# I'm not Lance!

*A Cancer Experience and
Survival Guide for Mere Mortals*

## By Scott P. Alcott

*For "Team Alcott":*
*Bernice, Gavin, and Zoe*

*You have given me a life worth*
*fighting very hard for*

# Acknowledgements

My parents, Robert and Margaret, and my brother, Kevin, who helped raise me and refused to lose me. Thanks, Kevin, for helpful editing advice!

My always supportive in-laws: Effie, Audrey, Clarice Chen and families.

Dr. Zalman Agus, Dr. David Agus, Mr. Joel Agus, and Dr. Joe Viggiano for helping me get diagnosed while no one else took my symptoms seriously.

Dr. Ara Chalian, Head and Neck Surgeon, Hospital University of Pennsylvania

Dr. Gary K. Schwartz, Chief of Melanoma and Sarcoma at Memorial Sloan Kettering Cancer Center, and the entire staff at MSKCC.

Didier Bellens and Belgacom for sticking with me when they didn't have to.

My wonderful friends and supporters from West Windsor-Plainsboro High, the University of Pennsylvania, AT&T, Ameritech, Belgacom and the gangs at Brussels, Oak Park, Princeton and Morristown.

The Johnson and Miller families for being inspiring role models.

Robert Kagan, for his friendship and for inspiring me to write.

Mimi Olsson, Bruce Shriver and the wonderful people for supporting each other on the "E-Sarcoma" Yahoo User Group and on Facebook.

Lance Armstrong, for leading the fight and supporting us all.

Nellie the cat, for living in the basement during my treatment!

# Contents

# Introduction

For my 40th birthday, I got stage four cancer. A small lump under my cheek turned out to be a rare, high-grade sarcoma. The doctor said I would need immediate surgery and a year of heavy radiation and chemotherapy, assuming I made it that long. I was told to "make arrangements".

The first copy of *It's Not About the Bike: My Journey Back to Life* came from my neighbor, a retired surgeon. If you haven't read it, that's Lance Armstrong's inspirational cancer book. A college friend sent me a second copy wrapped together with one of those bright yellow "Livestrong" bracelets that Lance's cancer foundation sells to raise money. When you get cancer, you get a lot of Lance stuff.

You probably know Lance's story by now but the details in his book are amazing. His testicular cancer spread everywhere including to his lungs and brain. He beat it against very long odds and went on to win the Tour de France seven consecutive times. Never a quitter, Lance just came out of retirement and is staring down the mountains again. More impressively (at least to me), he dated the singer, Sheryl Crow. He is objectively super-human! Lance routinely trains 180 days per year (in between racing events) and he likes to bike marathons before breakfast. Aerobically he has what's known as a $VO_2$ max of 83.8 ml per kilogram, which means he can sprint up a mountain and feel pretty much like you do when you're relaxing in front of the TV. His heart is 30% larger than yours is and it only beats about 32 times per minute.[1] He has unlimited endurance and at his peak, Lance had higher overall fitness, discipline, competiveness, and pain tolerance than anyone else in the world. Rumor is that Lance is also a candidate for governor of Texas someday. After reading his book, it was no surprise to me that this guy could beat cancer. I mean if not him, who can?

I work for a phone company. I'm 42 and married to Bernice, my freshman-year girlfriend. I'm not blessed with any special physical gifts. Like Lance, I ride a bike but usually around town with Bernice and the kids. I'm a bit soft at 6'1", 185 pounds, but normal enough I'd say. I don't smoke, do drugs, or drink excessively and I try to work out a few times a week when I can. For breakfast, I like the Princetonian Diner on Route 1 in New Jersey. You can get pumpkin pancakes, your choice of bacon or sausage, two eggs any style, juice and bottomless coffee for $11.99. I also have a relationship with Sheryl Crow. Her CD is in the Honda and my 8-year old daughter, Zoe, really likes her song, *Soak up the Sun*. My heart rate hits about 82 whenever Sheryl sings. I guess I'm no Lance.

Lance's book was immensely moving to me and his character and fighting spirit was inspiring. But could I measure up to him? He set the bar very high. I knew I didn't have Lance's bravery, stamina, pain

viii    I'm Not Lance!

tolerance, competitiveness, focus and physical gifts. I felt inadequate and ill-equipped for going into the same fight as him. Do I need to be like Lance Armstrong to beat this? Do people expect me to be that heroic, brave and committed? Is that why they gave me the book? It turns out that many do and some actually need you to be Lance-like. When you get cancer, you figure out quickly that the disease affects everyone around you, sometimes in unexpected ways.

I'm in remission now. Unlike Lance, no one is telling me I beat it yet. They scan me twice a year looking for tumor recurrence. Lance's life story is like a Hollywood movie with a triumphant conclusion. But all too often, it's not such a happy ending. I hope I beat this. I sure did some hard things to get this far.

All of us with cancer are fighting our own dramatic and heroic battles. We're hoping for our own come-from-behind victory like you see at the Tour de France—an against all odds type of thing. We also have many good people cheering us on, not always sure how to behave, what to say and how to cope.

This book is for patients and their supporters, whether you're new to the cancer community, in remission, or in the long term survivor stage. It's about what happens when regular people and their families find themselves in the very irregular situation that is cancer. It's an experience and survival guide for the rest of us.

# 1

## The "Open Door" Moment

"Suck it up," Lance told himself. By sheer will, he powered through coughing up blood, debilitating migraines and the painful swelling from cancer in his brain, lungs and testicle. "Of course I should have known that something was wrong with me," Lance recalls, but he was trained to not give into pain. His testicle was the size of an orange but he kept riding and training until he virtually collapsed from full-blown disease.

Mere mortals usually have a much less dramatic entry into the world of cancer. For many people, it's a routine or unrelated x-ray/CT scan that shows a "non-specific sub-centimeter nodule" on a lung or in breast tissue or maybe it's a small polyp on the colon. Often findings like this require waiting six months to see if the nodule changes over time because everyone has little scuffs and bumps of some kind.

Many others like me notice something very unspectacular and if we get it checked out, doctors tend to dismiss it. Cancer can present like a thousand benign things and worried patients are often made to feel like hypochondriacs when they have an odd sensation, a small pain, or a bump you can pinpoint but the doctor can't quite get a finger on. My cancer mainly affects athletic and otherwise healthy young boys and adolescents. Nearly everyone in our community was told it is "growing pains" or pulled muscles or something else benign. Other people with headaches, migraines, and eye pain are assumed to be stressed before a brain tumor is suspected and it's worse if you are otherwise healthy and not in a high-risk group.

Because I'm not Lance, I was kind of a baby about the small raised area I came upon while shaving. There's no way I could have an orange-sized testicle without panicking and even this little bump on my face concerned me! It was unusual and unlike Lance, I obsessed about it for several weeks. I did a little internet research and asked my wife if she could feel it too. Bernice finally suggested that I should go get it checked out so I could stop worrying about it.

I remember feeling ridiculous when I went to see my local family doctor. The waiting room was packed with obviously sick people, except for me. Having come directly from work, I was dressed sharp, buttoned up, and looked as great as I felt. I was planning a tennis match later that evening if the wait wasn't too long. I was totally asymptomatic, except for a small bump. Still too small to be visible, I probed around my face in the waiting room to be sure I could put a finger on it for the doctor. My wife and kids frequented this family doctor for the ear infections, rashes and check-ups that dominate the lives of young families. But I was the picture of health. I didn't have a single sick day in 20 years and I had never seen him before. When the door opened, I had the image of a medic on the front lines of a ground war—a guy who spent all day with acutely sick people in need of antibiotics, finger splints and shots. I felt like I was stealing from the needy sitting there on the examination table in a Brooks Brother's suit.

Without looking at me or introducing himself, the doctor went right to the chart where I checked "no" for everything they asked about symptoms, family history, recent illnesses and other medical problems. "So you have a bump somewhere?" he finally stammered. Now my practice would pay off and with confidence, I landed my index finger on the exact spot in one move. The doctor, however, couldn't find it. You have an advantage finding things in your own body because you can feel it from the finger side and the bump side simultaneously. After a few, "no, more to the left" kinds of interactions, he claimed to have found it. I'm still not sure if he was just throwing me a bone. I could see immediately I was done and he was going to get back to the sick people, but he tried to reassure me first.

"Look, little benign cysts and things happen all the time on the face and near the mouth. Nothing bad really ever happens there. You're young, fit, you don't smoke or have any risk factors and there's no family history of any problems. It's nothing and I'm sure. Keep an eye on it but don't worry about it." Translation, "Get out of my office you hypochondriac!" At least that's what I heard in my head. And trust me; I was happy for the news. I wasn't looking to have a problem.

Lethal cancers were not diagnosed or were misdiagnosed before death in 44% of cases, according to a 10-year retrospective study at a U.S. medical center.[2] That's because early stage cancer is often asymptomatic or presents like the aches, pains, bumps and twinges of everyday life. It's easy for patients and doctors alike to blow it off. You can't order an MRI for every head and body ache. And the doctor was right. My own internet research backed him up. Occasionally benign tumors around the salivary gland show up but rarely cancer, especially if you don't smoke or have other risk factors. It was a reasonable call.

I met many people in the cancer community like me, who had a feeling, some kind of 6th sense that something was wrong. I had never been a worrier but something in my head told me, against all assurances and data, that the small bump on my face was a problem. I left the doctor feeling not quite reassured. Many patients, like me, had trouble getting a doctor to take their problem seriously but a larger number acted like Lance, sucked it up, and ignored the pain themselves. In general, cancer patients often enter the community after having waited and endured doubt and skepticism about their symptoms for a long time. Because he is Lance Armstrong and because he waited until his symptoms were obviously an emergency, Lance didn't have to endure very much skepticism and teams started working for him in a flurry.

Unfortunately, for regular people, the waiting and uncertainty usually continues even after the situation deteriorates. My small bump didn't go away or remain stable; it started to become visible and hard. My eye started fluttering and twitching as nearby nerves were invaded by the growth. A return trip to the doctor graduated my bump from nothing to "probably nothing" and an MRI was ordered. They assumed a benign growth or cyst was the problem and because there are many nerves in the face, surgery was probable but just for cosmetic and nerve function reasons; still nothing serious. Maybe because I was considered lower risk, it took weeks to get the scan and an office appointment booked with a specialist. And when it was done, the stress wasn't resolved, just more questions and other tests to complete. The scans were consistent with everything from cat scratch fever to lymphoma but it was most likely a "benign pleomorphic neoplasm", whatever that meant. Suddenly my lump went from nothing to scary-sounding diseases and a needle biopsy was needed to get to the bottom of it all, which meant more waiting, another procedure and stress accumulating daily.

I still remember perfectly when a pair of young med students came in. With more brute force than technical grace, they bored and twisted a 6-inch long very fat needle directly into the lump on my face. They were 20-something females, attractively brainy in their lab coats, and clearly apologetic for the pain I was enduring. "Feels fine," I lied. They took the needle next door and immediately looked at it under a microscope. No more waiting. The moment of truth arrived.

Most of us don't learn about our cancer like Lance did with a dramatic collapse and advanced symptoms. For the rest of us, it's the "open door" moment that welcomes us to the community and my moment had arrived. There will be many of these "open door" moments during your battle but the first one is the hardest. You can tell right away when they come in. All they could tell from the biopsy was that it was malignant, high-grade and serious. I wasn't coughing up blood, having migraines and unlike Lance, I actually felt quite fine. But I wasn't fine. Surgery was scheduled immediately.

Bernice and I walked out startled. It's strange how you need to do routine things after such devastation. In a state of silent shock, we waited in line and did administrative things with the scheduling nurse. Then a silent long walk to the garage; the parking attendant had to be paid, keys retrieved, were we on level three or four? It was "tax day", April 2006, and I became a cancer statistic, an unwilling member of Lance's exclusive club.

# 2

## Measuring up to Lance

A man of action and speed, Lance got his diagnosis and was in surgery 7 a.m. the next day. It took me seven months from feeling my lump to getting someone to care and ultimately diagnose it. In one dramatic blink, Lance went from champion to the world's most famous cancer patient. "I have a tough constitution, and my profession taught me how to compete against long odds and big obstacles," Lance remarked. Not me. I cleaned off my desk and had a transition meeting with my replacement at work; and off I went without any experience or toolkit to fight such a battle.

Because I'm not Lance, I entered his club with a negative outlook and the presumption of defeat. A regular person feels subordinate to the infamous and all-powerful cancer. I'm not the world champion of anything but cancer is the #2 ranked killer in the world. And unlike the #1 killer (heart attacks), cancer defeats its opponents with a cruel, monotonous, slow and grinding punishment; death by torture. My opponent was a true monster with intimidating skills. For me it was like entering the ring against the mean and supremely trained boxer,

Mike Tyson, without any skill or prior training. Not only did I know such an opponent would kill me, I feared it would embarrass me in front of the crowd before putting me down. I saw myself being taken apart, revealed as inadequate, broken down, humiliated and crying for mercy in front of my kids; beaten to death by a laughing bully. Lance is a human being and like everyone, I'm sure he was scared and had doubts. But Lance knew he wouldn't go down humiliated and with loss of dignity. He knew he could take a punch, endure incredible pain and outmaneuver formidable adversaries. He was a winner and he was trained to compete with and beat other world champions. He intended to beat this world champion killer and knew he had the right to be in the ring with it and exchange punches head to head. "I'm determined to fight this disease," he said. "And I will win." I wasn't motivated when I read this. I just felt embarrassed to be in the same ring with a guy like Lance. I had no idea how to throw a knockout punch and felt half the man of Lance Armstrong. I didn't measure up.

As Lance's book kept arriving from well-wishers, the letters and phone calls also started coming in. "We know you're going to beat this!" was the typical refrain. "The main thing is to keep a good attitude, that's 90% of the battle." Really? It felt to me like everyone I knew was filing in, taking their seats next to the boxing ring for the big rumble, me the soft phone company guy against Tyson the trained man eater. "Just stay positive, we know you can beat this guy!" Are they kidding me? I'm going to be squashed.

I'm pretty sure Tyson would kill me regardless of my attitude and outlook and it turns out to be true with cancer too. The popular belief that positive attitude can help fight cancer has been debunked by a group of Australian specialists in 2008 who have proved a fighting spirit does not improve a patient's survival chances. The 10-year study found no correlation at all between outcome and levels of anxiety, depression, negativity, anger and feeling of hopelessness.[3] That's good news because I totally felt all of those negative emotions and apparently, that alone isn't going to kill me.

The study does admit that there are social benefits to having a good attitude and this is something cancer patients have always suspected. It's easier on everyone else if we enter that ring with a smile and hope; who wants to be around a guy who's sure he's going to die from a sustained, horrible public beating? Is that why we get multiple gift copies of Lance's book and the positive attitude encouragement? Is it a hint to suck it up like Lance and a plea for you to act like a world champion? Sometimes it feels that way when you get cancer and there is quite a bit of social pressure to be stoic, even heroic.

Of course, it's all positively motivated. What are people supposed to do, count you out before the bell even rings? They're standing with you and hoping you get off that lucky punch. They don't know what else to do. And that's one theme of this book. Cancer is a situation that causes certain rituals and behaviors because no other better behavioral option exists. I'm not pleading for behavior change by pointing out the uncomfortable truths behind these rituals. I am trying to deepen the understanding of what is going on in the heads of patients, friends, family, doctors and work colleagues so we can support each other better and avoid sending/receiving unintended wrong signals.

When you send me in the ring against Tyson and tell me you expect me to beat him by keeping a positive attitude, I feel conned and dealt with expediently and superficially. When you give me Lance's book as proof of hope, I feel more inadequate to the task than ever because his is a story of a superman, not a mortal man. I'm afraid to show you my doubt and talk with you about my fears because I'm told I shouldn't have those negative feelings and indulging them can kill me (the positive attitude myth). I'm not Lance and I need a sign that you understand that but still think I can win the fight.

Everyone else has unspoken hushed needs too and cancer etiquette prevents us from openly talking about what your family and friends need. They're expected to support the sick patient and often their very complex needs are left unattended. Turns out everyone is expected to suck it up and act heroically during cancer. It's even true for your doctor. After dealing with cancer end-to-end for a while now, I have a sense of grand theater, role-playing, ritual and activity put in place as a mass coping strategy for the entire community. There are many head fakes in such a system and because things are not as they appear to be, wrong steps and misunderstandings can pop up.

Newly diagnosed patients, their families and the medical community can benefit by knowing what simmers underneath to avoid head fakes, to send better and more clear signals, and to work the giant project of cancer management more efficiently and with less wasted energy. The successful day-to-day management of cancer requires a thorough understanding of the stakeholders in your community, their biases, needs, attitudes and requirements.

Lance was a model patient and he raised the bar for everyone around him. He assembled a world-class medical team and inspired his supporters to be realistic but optimistic, like him. This became a virtuous circle with patient, doctor, and friends all lifting each other. It's harder when regular people like me get cancer. Our doubts, imperfections, inefficiencies and fear infect the entire community. I wondered if I could close the gap with Lance.

# 3

## Taking Punches

Bernice cried when they wheeled me into the operating room. My brother, Kevin, dropped everything and flew in from Chicago and my parents made the trek from North Carolina to be there in west Philadelphia. They must have all known what had not yet occurred to me. In the blur of a cancer diagnosis, it was actually the first time it hit me how badly this could all go. I kept my composure and went in ready to face whatever was to come. Some kind of coping mechanism kicks in at times like this and I was strangely calm. It was ice cold and blinding bright in there, all business. The surgeon and anesthesiologist bantered with me, I guess to cut the edge off the moment. My eye had started to twitch in the days before the surgery. The doctor felt this was because the cancer had spread to nearby nerves and from there, to god knows where. There was no way of telling how far the surgery would have to go. Before they put me under, I told the doctor that if it came to it, he should choose getting the cancer out ahead of preserving my looks or function. I knew I could lose half my face, maybe even my eye and my jaw, but I had young kids and needed to be aggressive.

When you get cancer, you have difficult calls to make. He understood with a nod and I was out.

I was surprised how big the scar was. It ran from my collarbone to my temple. I could no longer feel my right ear and a large dent was where my cheek used to be. My ear was asymmetric now, apparently having been pulled off with a skin flap and sewn back on after the tumor was excised. I was disfigured and still had dried blood in between the surgical stitches. The good news was the cancer seemed localized. The tumor was small, about two centimeters, and it was just lying in the soft tissue of my cheek not connected to anything especially important. There was no sign of spreading into the lymph nodes and he didn't need to take my eye, jaw or bone structure. For safety reasons, he took out part of the nearby parotid gland, clipped some nerves that had been touching the tumor and cut away as much surrounding soft tissue he could to get the widest surgical margins possible. The surgeon was pleased with his work and was somewhat surprised that I could still smile, blink and control my face given the nerve cuts. I wasn't pretty but I was alive and it was a lot better than it could have been.

Unfortunately, this was not the end. I scanned clear of any other tumors and something called a PET scan was able to tell that no scant cancer cells were even floating around; at least not ostensibly. But the good news ended there. Pathology determined I had a rare cancer called Ewing's Sarcoma. There are only about 300 diagnosed per year in the U.S., most cases are in children and most are in the bone, especially in the leg and pelvis. The odds of a 40-year-old adult getting the soft tissue variety in the face were astronomical. I could more easily have won the lottery…twice. Unfortunately, this cancer almost always does something called "occult metastases" which means it spreads microscopically from the original tumor throughout the body without being detectable by our current technology. I would soon have multiple tumors in the lungs and vital organs and it would kill me if I didn't get in front of the cancer; I was quickly transferred to a sarcoma specialist.

The doctor immediately worked up a treatment plan. I was scheduled for nearly a year of aggressive chemotherapy and enough radiation to shame Chernobyl. I was given a coin-toss prognosis--a 50% shot at making it five years, assuming I survived the treatment. My oncologist thought this was very encouraging. In his line of work it is. In my line of work, 50% success rate gets you fired.

Because I'm not Lance, I pretty much quit on myself at this point. I wasn't up for the drama. Fussing for a year with pills and doses, appointments and injections, nausea and radiation sickness, baldness and toxicity... for a coin toss shot? I doubted I could do it mentally or physically. This disease hits less than one in a million. I felt like beating such a thing was like trying to out-run lightning. It felt predestined. Maybe Lance could stare down such a mountain but I never did anything impossible before. No, this was bigger than me. I was quite sure it would win. Chemo was scheduled to begin in two weeks and for me, it was the beginning of the end.

*Chemotherapy*

My instincts were correct. Chemotherapy was the beginning of the end, literally. It's a treatment strategy that attempts to kill the cancer by nearly killing you. It's like when firemen set a controlled blaze to prevent a larger forest fire from spreading out of control. And trust me; you are burned with this strategy.

Memorial Sloan Kettering Cancer Center (MSKCC) is one of the oldest and best cancer hospitals in the world. MSKCC does chemo in several locations in New York and New Jersey. The newer ones try to model a first class international flight experience. The waiting room resembles the executive frequent flyer lounge at a major airport. When you arrive, attractive hostesses greet you. After presenting your exclusive "member card" at the desk, you are recognized and addressed by name by all of the staff. "Mr. Alcott, we'll be doing vitals and a CBC before inviting you back for chemo. Please have a seat and we'll be with you shortly." There are comfortable leather sofas casually strewn about a modern, open-plan room. There are coffee and juice bars, pretzels and snacks for the taking, newspapers, magazines, flat screen TV's, internet stations and a spa-like soothing fountain.

Of course, there are the sick people. You start to recognize the regulars—they're on the same cycle as you and you'll be seeing them for a long time. You notice the ones that don't seem to be tolerating well and you don't speak about the ones that don't come back. You're sorry when a newbie with hair shows up in the lobby unaware of what awaits him. Business is good, there's a newbie every week. If your blood is not too toxic from the last treatment, you get invited back to the treatment room to get your next round of poison. Now you're in the first class seat kitted out with a personal video machine, reclining lounger, and team of first class attendants.

There's gallows humor everywhere in the Chemo Room. Everyone tries to act like it's a routine thing. You joke with the nurses and say hi to the people you recognize. Someone asks what the specials are today and they offer you nausea meds and steroids in a little bowl like it's an appetizer. The staff knows you and you are intimate without actually knowing each other. Everyone tells you how good you look and you try and act like it's just another day at the office. It's a creepy place trying to seem normal.

When your meds come up from the lab freshly mixed, everything turns serious. There's a failsafe procedure like in the movies when the President orders the nuclear strike. Suddenly I'm a stranger. There's a hush and stern faces. Surgical gloves are on now and it's all business. I need to  identify myself by saying and spelling my name and giving my birthday in front of witness nurses. The first nurse reads off the drug name and dosage from the label on the drip bag. The other one verifies it with the doctor's order sheet reading back the same information. "Doxorubicin, 72 milligrams per meter squared, IV drip over 2 hours. Check." The bags they are holding in gloved hands are lethal and they kill. Mix up a patient and someone dies. You can't mix certain drugs and you can't pass certain cumulative doses. There can be no mistakes.

Chemotherapy is programmed cell death. They tap a vein and pump in toxic compounds designed to find and kill fast growing cells. You literally die, or at least a sizeable percent of your cells die during the process and you can feel that part of your body going. When I'm asked what it's like, I say it's like dying and being reborn every 21 days—a physical and mental death followed by the euphoria of simply being alive again… just briefly before it all starts again.

When the vincristine hit my veins, I could feel it course through my system in a second and hit my brain. Instantly I went from witty conversation to being gone, awake but flat-lined, a zombie with a fried brain. When a cat dies, it goes off somewhere safe and dark and does it alone. The fractional death of chemo was like that for me, something intensely personal and private. I couldn't bear to let anyone but Bernice see my partial death. Family and friends don't understand this. Many want to come and support you and be with you while you are being killed. It was too heavy having company while I died every day. It was too much energy to try to act normal, strong and reassuring. I felt the burden of looking after the watchers and couldn't carry it. Lance was different. He had a large group of rotating supporters who would come and watch him compete with pain and death. I suppose he was trained that way. His entire life was to perform for crowds as he took on incredible pain and impossible physical challenges. He must have been more confident than me to manage it all.

The wine-colored doxorubicin was the hardest to tolerate and lethal too. Its toxicity cumulates and stays with you permanently. If it gets on your skin, it would burn a hole so they're careful to make sure the needle is fully in a vein where the rapid circulation keeps the burn moving. You can only do a cumulative total of 550 mg of "Dox" before toxic heart failure becomes a very big risk. I got right up to that line. In total I did a cocktail of five different chemos usually for 8 hours per day for a full week and then cooked, experienced massive cellular death, recovered and did it again every three weeks for half a year. In support, I was on four different nausea control meds, steroids and I injected myself in the stomach every cycle with a miracle drug called Neulasta® that replenishes white blood cells. Without Neulasta, you can die on chemo from the common cold. Neulasta is $1,200 a shot if you inject yourself and $2,000 if the hospital does it; and it is worth every penny.

Everyone on chemo has a different experience. There are different drugs depending on your disease, different doses and frequencies. Everyone has different metabolisms and abilities to tolerate different compounds. Some people can't do it. Many fall off cycle and have to miss important doses because their body can't take the toxicity. Some people die from the chemo itself or from the infections that it enables. I joked that my long line of Irish relatives and my hard training at Murphy's Tavern during college gave me a leg up as I tolerated it all pretty well, relatively speaking. Painful mouth sores, lost hair, convulsions, constipation, fatigue, and steroidal mood swings were part of a day's work; so was the sterility and the destruction of heart muscle, bone mass, and blood cells. Getting the chemo was the easy part although finding a vein and being poked a thousand times started to get harder as all the good veins collapsed. The truly hard part came a few days later when the cells dying in my body started to accumulate.

You could smell the poison coming out of my pores no matter how many times I showered; and I could taste it—stronger every day. Cells in your mouth and esophagus die quickly from chemo and you get painful lesions making it difficult to eat and swallow. Your urine resembles an acid puddle at a toxic waste dump. As your white and red blood cells die off, you get fatigued and feel shocky. You can't eat fresh fruit or salads because without white blood cells, any uncooked food could pass bacteria or a virus that you would have no defenses against. Purell® became a staple in my house as everyone hand-sanitized constantly. Bernice disinfected doorknobs, light switches and all surfaces to help keep me safe.

When the Neulasta shot kicked in, I would get massive bone pain everywhere as it pushed white blood cells out of my bone marrow via a trick of genetic engineering. I looked forward to this pain as it signaled the "turn"—the end of cell death and the start of recovery. As each day improved, euphoria began to set in. It felt like springtime and rebirth. During this recovery cycle over the year of my treatment, I: invented new business ideas and applied for a U.S. patent; put a bid on three houses that were for sale (and lost them all to competitors); wrote songs and poetry; went fishing, kayaking, took road trips, went to parties; and re-mastered the art of throwing a curve ball. There is a burst energy that comes with rebirth and I didn't waste those moments! But like a prisoner on a weekend release program, it would end abruptly—back to the cell. It was time to start dying again. And the whole cycle would repeat.

*Radiation Therapy*

Lance and I both did surgery and chemo but unfortunately, I had an additional torture to endure that he was lucky enough to escape. Chemotherapy's main job is to chase down cancer cells that are floating around anywhere in your bloodstream, tissue and organs. Radiation has a different objective. It's usually targeted and focused on a specific spot of concern. In my case, there just wasn't enough tissue in the face to surgically remove a large block with "wide margins" around the tumor. That meant microscopic cancer cells at the border of the surgical cut could have survived and this was bad for my prognosis.

Sending high-energy radiation all around my tumor area was kind of a mop-up strategy and I needed to do this in addition to the chemotherapy. Radiation also kills good cells along with the bad ones and it does damage that cumulates. Like a gunshot, there is an entry and exit wound caused by the radioactive beam and things in the field of treatment are affected. Radiation to the head and neck is hard to tolerate and dangerous; it is a precision exercise. A custom fiberglass mask is made to the exact contour of your head and with screws attached, you are bolted down to a table to prevent any movement during treatment. It is so tight that you could sneeze violently and not be able to move a millimeter. Three permanent tattoos, small dots on your face and chest, help the technician precisely triangulate your position under the machine so the energy beam can be perfectly directed by computer.

Like with chemo, there are safety and security procedures for radiation therapy to avoid mix-ups. There is a digital image of my face on the machine's control panel that acts as an electronic key to associate me with my treatment profile. Once I identify the image as me in front of two witnesses who agree, the computer loads the exact energy, duration and shape of the beam that is designed specifically for me and we're off for another treatment. Once again, it's a first class flight complete with valet parking, a modern lounge and staff that treat you like the frequent flyer that you are. This flight costs over $1,500 for 10 minutes and the machine is billed out for 12 hours per day. You have the same technician every day and you report to the very same machine for your exclusive private session. Membership has its privileges!

You feel nothing when the radiation blast hits you. The machine is on a robotic arm and it changes positions as it attacks the treatment area from different angles. I needed to do this every weekday for seven weeks—34 treatments in all. It starts slowly at first. You get a sunburn kind of sensation after a few days. By the end, you're like a hamburger that was put in a microwave too long—cooked from the inside out until it's desiccated. My skin became inflamed, purple, and very painful. My tongue and mouth were burned and filled with lesions. I lost all sense of taste and food became unappetizing, even nauseating. For me, I found radiation worse than the chemotherapy. It was a marathon without breaks. Its damage accumulated every day without the rebirth cycles that came with chemo.

Losing the ability to taste anything is much more traumatic than you would expect. I was never more aware of how much life is centered on eating or preparing food and going out to restaurants...all of which became painful and unpleasant to me. To this day, even though my ability to taste has recovered, certain foods are still nauseating because I associate them with this time. Radiation also meant no sun exposure—even to untreated parts of the body. The floppy hats, oversized dark glasses, and baggy clothes made me feel isolated and eccentric while others were in the pool or at the little league game.

When I returned from my first treatment, Bernice unveiled a poster on the wall, a graph with 34 increments sloping up to the right to show the accumulation of my work, all of it still to come. A tiny single box was colored green to represent completing the first step of the mountain that was in front of me. Every session, the kids would shade another bar to mark my progress and keep me focused on the finish line. It was a grueling slog. I (literally) took the heat and finished all 34 treatments. It took every inch of endurance I could muster, like a marathon when you collapse at the finish line. I was done but the pain and damage were still accumulating, like a piece of meat that still cooks after it leaves the oven.

The hospital staff gave me my mask after the final treatment. It was like bringing a piece of my prison home with me. I didn't want to see it again; it was an object of cruelty and torture so I tossed it without ceremony. Unfortunately, I wasn't done yet. Chemotherapy was paused because combining it with radiation was too lethal. I had three weeks off before starting another four months of chemo poisoning but this time with a different cocktail. The doctor warned me that I had done the easy part. This cocktail was harder, very few people could tolerate it consistently, and few tried to do it all outpatient. He also knew I was weaker and broken down by the months of surgery, chemo and radiation that came before. It was too bad, my hair just started to come back after having been off chemo a few months; just a tease. It wasn't long before I was pale, sickly, bald and smelling like chemicals again.

*We're now boarding our first class passengers*

A funny thing about cancer is that you get busy dealing with it all. The activity of treating cancer is pre-occupying and for many, it becomes the focus rather than disease itself. In my case, the treatment certainly was more acutely risky and present than the actual disease. Strangely, all the appointments, screenings, lab tests, injections and pills helped me cope a little. The side effects, pain of the treatment, and the management of the side effects distracted from the unthinkable problem at the root of all of this activity. In the thick of it all, I stopped focusing on my readiness to fight cancer. I had things to do and it quickly became a job with a million appointments and details to manage.

I was now aboard the cancer plane and was starting to become an experienced frequent flyer. For my own self-image, I bumped myself up a notch. I had just completed surgery, months of chemo and radiation—that's three rounds in the ring with the world's meanest killer, and I was still standing. So were many of the brave people I met along the way in chemo and radiation rooms. When the last radiation treatment was done, they did a full body scan looking for tumors. They wanted a baseline before restarting chemo. All remained clear; there was no evidence of recurring cancer. I thought to myself, "Maybe I'm not Lance, but I can take a punch too." Score one for the mortals.

# 4

## F.U.D.

When I first got my cancer diagnosis, I felt like a convicted criminal. How long was my sentence, would I be incarcerated, am I allowed to leave the state? I didn't understand if the disease itself would debilitate me and I wondered if the doctors and treatment protocol would shackle me to a hospital bed, preventing me from working and living. I didn't know the penalty for my crime. I wanted some kind of authority figure, a "cancer warden", to read me my rights.

Once again, it was different for Lance. He didn't see himself as a subordinate to cancer. He took charge of his situation and wrote his own rules. Not only did he leave the state, he actually went on a national search and put himself in charge of choosing the right treatment plan and doctor team. I was so scared by my "conviction" that I wasn't even sure if I was allowed to go home! My instinct was to go to my room and wait for instructions. There was an enormous amount of fear, uncertainty, and doubt (F.U.D.). I had seen cancer dramatized on TV and in the movies and I knew some others who had a wide range of experiences. What would come next?

When you get your diagnosis, you quickly learn the particulars of your case and what's expected. But there are some important myths to break and some common experiences that apply widely.

*Is cancer painful?*

I'm frequently asked how the cancer felt and most people assume it is painful and present. Cancer can cause pain because it invades tissues and compresses nerves. But, only about one-third of cancer patients in active therapy have significant pain.[4] Most patients, especially in early stages, have no significant pain and may be totally without symptoms at all. In my case, I could see and feel a mass under my skin but there was no feeling of "having cancer". As time went on, the mass invaded nearby nerves and created twinges and fluttering around my eye but that was incidental and only a fleeting annoyance. I often tell people that cancer, for me, was physically a non-event, while treatment for cancer was a giant physical challenge and much more present.

*Does everyone have to do chemotherapy and radiation?*

Combination therapy refers to the use of surgery, chemotherapy, and radiation as a three-prong strategy for fighting cancer. This is standard protocol for certain cancers like mine; other times the situation may warrant all or some mix of those strategies. When cancer has spread beyond a local zone, chemotherapy may be needed to find cancer cells wherever they may be hiding. When chemo is used after surgery, it is called "adjuvant therapy". Chemo can also be used as a "neo-adjuvant" strategy to shrink tumors before surgery making removal easier and safer. If a tumor is situated in between nerves or in hard to reach areas, radiation may be useful because the energy beam can reach the tumor with less collateral damage than surgery. In many cases, surgery or radiation alone is the standard protocol for cancer, especially cancers found in early stages. It's important to know that many types and stages of cancer can be managed without combination therapy and many require no chemotherapy treatment at all.

*Are you always sick?*

According to a recent study, cancer patients fear chemotherapy more than dying.[5]  The profound side effects of nausea and sickness are an overwhelming prospect for most people. It's important to know that enormous progress has been made in making this awful treatment more tolerable and the gains are very real.

Many people today tolerate their chemotherapy treatment very well with little incidence of nausea, vomiting and sickness. This is new and it's all due to breakthrough developments in a class of drugs called "antiemetics" that stop nausea symptoms before they start. Vomiting and nausea are a natural protection mechanism that your body uses to eliminate poison in your system. When you eat spoiled food, consume too much alcohol, or have a virus in your stomach, sensors notice the toxins and send a signal to your brain which, in turn, triggers nausea and vomiting to eliminate the culprit. It's the same with chemotherapy. Your stomach senses the chemo as a toxin that should be eliminated and literally tries to push it out. Antiemetics block the receptors in the stomach and the brain essentially disconnecting the biological communication chain that causes vomiting. It really works.

You certainly won't feel great but many patients can expect to avoid nausea, vomiting and sickness altogether. I did a wide range of chemotherapy drugs known to be especially debilitating and at high dosages for a long duration. In nearly a year of treatment, I never vomited once and never felt nauseous.  By controlling this side effect, higher doses are being given today (still without nausea) and more medicine means greater chances to beat the cancer.

There are, of course, no guarantees. Some chemotherapy drugs cause nausea more than others and some people can simply tolerate toxins better than others. There is no cure-all but the days of guaranteed sickness are over. Sometimes the doctors need trial and error to determine which antiemetics or which combination of them works best for you. Typically, I was given a Zofran® pill, a steroid, and an intravenous drip of Aloxi® thirty minutes before chemo infusion began. I then took Emend® daily after the injections were completed. The specific drugs used for nausea control depend on the chemo you are doing and how well you tolerate it.

There is also evidence that your relative ability to tolerate chemotherapy roughly approximates your ability to tolerate alcohol, with light drinkers having a rougher time. If you get hangovers easily, chemo may have a similar effect. Once again, I thank my long line of Irish relatives for giving me an edge on chemo!

*What about all those needles?*

Cancer patients face the prospect of constant injections and needles. When you get cancer, this does become an important part of your life and you do get used to it. Injections for chemotherapy are never ending but that's only part of the problem. Cancer means constant blood tests to check for disease indicators and to see if chemo has done too much damage to platelets, red and white blood cells. Cancer also means recurring radiological PET, CT and MRI scans, which require injections of iodine and/or radioactive isotopes to be read effectively. Finally, there are the magical shots of Epogen® or Neulasta to help replace the lost blood cells ravaged by chemotherapy.

There's a multiplier-effect with all these injections; the trauma makes veins collapse so 2-3 pokes are needed every time to find a "bleeder".

There are some tricks to lessen the burden and many cancer patients consider a needle saved a personal victory. Patients who face extensive chemotherapy simply get a "port" put in. A port is a device inserted under the skin near the collarbone with a catheter on one end connecting into a vein. The other end has a "door" and once installed, no injections are needed for chemotherapy; it's simply pumped in through the open door. When treatment is done for good, the port is removed. It's considered minor surgery and many patients find it's a godsend eliminating one of the miseries of chemotherapy. It's not risk-free as the port can sometimes become infected or blocked and some can find it awkward feeling. In spite of lengthy treatment, I did all my chemo without a port although it became harder later as veins collapsed.

Another strategy for reducing injections is a simple idea, but it is often overlooked. Hospitals have departments and shifts that may have no idea what other departments or shifts need to do. In the early days of my treatment, I would go to one floor and have a blood test (prick #1); an hour later I'd be getting a CT scan of the head on floor 5 (prick #2); and 2 hours after that a whole body CT scan (prick #3). As I became more experienced, I managed all of that to become just one needle. By telling the first technician that I had several other procedures still to come, he inserted a "heparin lock" which is essentially a place holder for the later injections. It's a simple vial filled with saline, stuck in to your vein, and taped over with medical wrap; it lets the next technician use the same pin prick for later procedures. Think of it as a temporary port. I started to schedule my procedures intelligently to conserve injections. Since I had chemo sessions several days in a row, many times the nurses would let me go home with a heparin lock in place to avoid a new injection the next day. I estimate that I saved 30%-40% of injections with these simple tricks.

*Does everyone lose their hair?*

Hair loss is one of the most visible signs of cancer and people often find it the most traumatic moment of the battle. It's not just aesthetic, for many people it's a physical underline, a billboard that advertises your sickness. Going bald is a scarlet letter that classifies you as sick to others. People assume it's worse for women because many men are already bald and sometimes fashionably so. But "cancer baldness" is different in a way that signals illness; there is the sickly pallor and an absence of eyebrows and stubble that gives you away.

Hair loss is not automatic with cancer. Patients who are lucky enough to avoid chemo or radiation to the head can escape this problem entirely. For patients who do have more extensive treatment, hair loss can vary considerably, even for people taking the same drugs. Some people lose no hair, others lose only hair on the scalp, and others, like me, lose every single hair wherever it may have been. It just depends. In my case it came out in clumps a few weeks into the chemotherapy treatment. I could literally grab a fistful of hair and pull it out with no pain or resistance. Later, it just dumped in sheets while I was showering.

There are a few practical tips for managing the physical and psychological impact of impending hair loss. Before starting chemo, I cut my hair very short. This gave me (and my social circle) a chance to experience my hair loss in steps and it made the ultimate baldness less traumatic. This can be especially helpful for women who may have had long hair for a lifetime; taking a first, small interim step can be a bit of a soft landing. Having shorter hair also made the clean-up more manageable when the clumps started coming out.

Another helpful tip is to buy a good electric shaver because the worst look is when most hair falls out but clumps and strands remain. When it starts to go, buzz it off fast. My razor failed midway during the task and I was left with a half head of hair while Bernice ran around looking for a replacement! Women and men alike should prepare for this moment in advance by buying bandanas, hats and wigs if desired.

A final good lesson is to take passport and driver's license photos while you have hair, before these documents expire. I learned about this the hard way and now have a bald man who doesn't look very much like me emblazoned on these documents. I've had difficulty boarding airplanes, clearing immigration, and I often need to explain in public that I'm a cancer patient. The photos are a stressful reminder that can remain for years. Advance planning can make a major difference!

*Will you waste away and lose weight?*

The image many people have of cancer patients is bald, pale and thin as a rail. People used to waste away on chemotherapy because of widespread nausea and vomiting that usually came with the therapy. It was difficult to eat and keep food down. As discussed earlier, phenomenal gains in nausea control have made this much less of a problem; most patients today have an easier time maintaining their weight. But there are other challenges to overcome.

Cancer that is found in the gastro-intestinal track of course can directly impede the body's ability to absorb nutrients and process food. This can cause dangerous levels of weight loss and malnutrition and is a medical emergency as serious as the cancer itself. Patients with these conditions will be helped with specific protocols, including intravenous fluids and nutrients, in order to maintain weight.

The biggest challenge for maintaining weight is fighting the energy burn that comes from cancer treatment. Radiation and chemo do serious (intended) damage and the body expends enormous energy taking that punishment and even more energy is needed to replace cells destroyed by the therapy. Radiation and chemotherapy can cause dehydration and if not replaced, "water loss" from your cells will also cause weight loss. Unless calories and fluids are increased, the extra workload of treatment will cause weight loss and physical fatigue even without vomiting or sickness. I deliberately doubled my normal calories during treatment but maintained the exact same weight throughout, which shows how much energy is burned by treatment.

Cancer and cancer treatment are stressful physically and mentally and you often lose sleep and expend energy worrying. This also adds a new load to your energy reserves and can contribute to wasting. Many cancer patients benefit from relaxation exercises, meditation, counseling, and moderate exercise to burn stress.

Strangely, some patients actually gain weight during cancer treatment. Many treatment protocols include steroids and other drugs that build mass and retain water and others get huge appetites from the extra work they are doing. A few extra pounds can offer a well needed reserve during cancer treatment so abandon the vanity and let it come!

*Are you admitted to the hospital the entire time?*

Outpatient cancer treatment has become the preferred method for patients in the last five years and it is growing fast. This is because better drugs limit treatment side effects including nausea, neutropenia (low white blood cell count) and fever. It's now more cost effective, comfortable, and safer for the patient to go home and sleep in one's own bed after a day of chemotherapy than staying in the hospital overnight. Satellite clinics and full service "outpatient centers" are often conveniently located at major hospitals but also in dedicated care centers in residential areas. 24-hour communication and shift doctors provide around-the-clock support and remote patient monitoring. Radiation therapy is also done outpatient with recurring short appointments in a "park and go" setting. Unless your cancer is in advanced stages or requires specialized treatment, there is a good chance you can do your treatment outpatient.

Outpatient doesn't mean "free to go". You stagger out of the chemo room in a daze at the end of your torture and are in no condition to drive or take public transportation. You must have a companion to support you end-to-end when you are outpatient. You need to avoid crowds and sources of potential infection and you must be on red alert for signs of fever, shock, toxicity or infection. You cannot be in your cabin at the lake, on an airplane, or road trip if any of those problems develop; go back to your care facility without delay. You are released after treatment sessions when you are outpatient, but you are on a short tether!

When you get home, you need to control your environment to avoid sickness and infection. That means having your own bathroom, lots of hand washing, and elimination of unnecessary visitors—which can be the hardest. Supporters may want to visit outpatients with toddlers and new babies to raise spirits with new life—unfortunately, little ones also bring runny noses and dirty diapers which can be a real threat to chemo patients. Visiting pets may also need quarantine.

The hardest part of outpatient therapy is the added stress of travel and commuting to and from a very difficult treatment. Driving in a car for any length of time during chemo can be a rough way to start the morning. Still, for many, it's worth it. A hospital is a terrible place to stay and it's hard to get rest and relax there. Retreating to the comforts of home is a welcome alternative after a hard day's battle. For many people, it's the best choice.

*Can I still work or go to school?*

If your work or school can be done remotely by computer and telephone during flexible or reduced times, it's possible to work while getting treated for cancer. It might even be advisable if it can keep your mind and spirit sharp. I was lucky enough to have an employer who replaced me day-to-day with an "interim" manager but kept me officially on active status. They let me work when I felt able and I often did it remotely from home or the hospital. I was very lucky. Many patients are quickly declared "inactive" and get put on disability. Still, cancer treatment is a full-time job with many appointments and unplanned events and it takes a great mental and physical toll. Work that requires physical activity, interaction with the public, or committed regular shifts can be hard because of the risks of treatment and variability in treatment schedules. With little control over your schedule and interval periods of sickness and unavailability, it can be very challenging to work.

*Can I exercise?*

It's a great idea physically and mentally to keep fit and engage in moderate exercise. Always check first with your doctor but in general, it's recommended with common sense limits.

*What about sex?*

This is also something to discuss with your doctor, especially if the cancer directly affects sexual organs. Because sex can increase the chance of passing or developing an infection, care is needed especially during the chemo interval when white blood cells are low. Because chemotherapy and other medicines are excreted in body fluids, doctors advise taking appropriate measures to prevent exposing your partner to those chemicals during active treatment.

*Pardon the crime*

I found every step of cancer management became easier with experience. Once I learned the rhythm of my body and how it responded to chemo and radiation, I was less anxious and my physical and mental state improved. It takes just a couple of lab visits, scans and treatment cycles before you learn the ropes and suddenly, it's not as scary as it seemed when you were getting started. Cancer treatment is unpleasant but for me it was tolerable. I kept living a reasonably normal life during my battle and many do exactly the same. We've reached the point where patients should no longer fear the treatment more than the disease itself. The caricature of a bald and sickly patient is history. It turns out a cancer diagnosis wasn't a conviction at all and there never was a crime. Yes, it's a serious illness and the treatment is incredibly hard; but today, even mere mortals can hope to live a full life during the battle. Fear of the unknown is worse than the reality.

# 5

## Life in Cancerville, U.S.A

Cancer is a community disease; everyone around you gets it too. In effect, my friends, family and work colleagues unwittingly moved into a new community, Cancerville, U.S.A. This is a place with its own rules, traditions and social norms. It's a bad neighborhood with good people trying to get by. Many are trying to cope themselves and others are trying to help you cope with life on "cancer row". It's heavy interacting with someone who could be dying and it's hard to maintain the vigil. What do you say in Cancerville when you bump into the guy who is scarred, bald and obviously very sick? By the time I started second round chemo, I was a very well known citizen in Cancerville.

But eventually, even the good people in Cancerville have to go back to being happy, living life's normal routines and having fun. It can be awkward doing that when the struggling guy enters the party. People start to feel guilty about "getting back to normal" while someone they love is waging a painful and epic battle for their life…but they can't be in a constant mourning mode. That's not good for them or you. Social dynamics are totally screwed up by cancer and so are the practical and transactional things. Treatment means you are exposed, open to infections, needing to be isolated or just plain sick. Being a cancer patient means your calendar is fully booked with more urgent things to do, even on Christmas Day or during your cousin's big wedding. You are unpredictable, unreliable and can't make long-range plans. You are in limbo while everyone else's lives continue and eventually when "mourning mode" stops, a small part of everyone around you wants, needs or expects your life to normalize too. No one, not even the most empathetic and close supporter, can remain in a crisis with you at the level of crisis you are having in your own head.

Cancer is a community disease but no one except other cancer patients can really relate. Healthy people reading this will disagree believing they fully understand, relate and can approximate the physical and mental situation of their loved one. But cancer patients who are total strangers know that's not quite true. We see each other every day in the chemo room and with a glance make an instant connection that says, "I know". And we do. And we're glad that you don't.

*Thank you, kind stranger*

Bizarrely, it is the strangers and more fringe associates in Cancerville who seem most able to surprise with random acts of humanity and kindness. Plainly bald and sick but interested in a sturdy looking Volvo, the hard-edged used-car salesman shook his head at me, confided that it was a lemon, and sold me a reliable and less expensive Honda instead. He even offered to buy it back at cost when I was done using it for my treatment. "I'd like to help if I can," he said. When I signed the lease for an apartment to be nearer to family support and my hospital, the landlord, a tree of a man named Bill, gave me a hug and volunteered to drive me into New York for my treatments. He decided to cut the lawn for me every week too. As the word got out, people from my far past (including people I fired!) wrote long, hand-written letters and sent thoughtful gifts encouraging me; others from high school suddenly re-emerged with care and support. I've been approached by perfect strangers in a shopping mall, hugged, and encouraged. Everyone has a family member, a friend, or a co-worker going through something terrible and they empathize with you and it's sincere.

Lance writes beautifully about the angelic professional strangers who save your life. The chemo nurses, the radiation technicians, and your oncologist's secretary routinely make family out of a rotating community of often dying people. It's amazing how they adopt you into their care and empathy like family and you realize they are doing it for hundreds of needy people. It must take a terrible toll on them giving their heart to so many sick people, so many of whom don't make it.

*The near and the dear ones*

It's harder for people closer to you. The strangers have the luxury of caring about you without having to live with or own the horror. Your parents, wife, children, in-laws and closest friends have a different reality. The people close to you are sick too and need much the same support. But they don't get the goodwill of strangers. They have to go to work or school, pay the bills, help you and no one gives them medicine to get better. Often cancer patients can boost themselves up for brief visits from distant friends but it's harder to sustain day after day in front of closer family. Sometimes we try less hard around the people closest to us because we are more at ease and not on guard. Sometimes sick people are lousy to the people closest to them and more comfortable showing the temper, frustration and bitterness that can come with cancer. This can be hard on family who feel they are carrying a big load themselves and supporting you with hard work at the same time.

My mother, father, brother, Bernice and the kids were there for me every step of the way and variously played the role of psychologist, medical researcher, insurance negotiator, scan and office visit supporter, chauffeur, and even janitor, just to name a few. They didn't always get back the most considerate "me" and it's true in most cancer families. Holidays especially bring out the "cancer grouch" it seems!

I was given a chemo respite on Thanksgiving Day, a well needed reprieve to nurse my nausea and shock. For me it was a well deserved break and I assumed everyone understood that the normal holiday celebrations were cancelled that year. When I learned that the entire family wanted to go forward as usual, I was offended and angry; don't they get my situation? It turns out they did completely. My family had a clearer state of mind than I did. They understood that I would regret giving away the magic moments in life, especially when they could be my last. It wasn't easy for my mom and dad, nearly 70 at this time, to drive during holiday traffic for a thousand miles to be with me for this celebration. But I can still see the photo in my mind. We were all dressed up, laughing, and slightly embarrassed by our appetite-- three generations beating the crap out of the unlimited Thanksgiving buffet at the Hyatt Regency. "We bankrupted this place!" said Gavin, as he flashed a gap-toothed grinned before wiping gravy off his face with the sleeve of his best white dress shirt. Somehow, I wasn't sick anymore. They were right to go ahead with the holiday.

With that experience in hand, I decided that if I was going to die during my treatment year, my kids were not going to remember me as negative, grouchy and defined by my sickness. And that changed everything for me. I did 8 hours of chemo, walked out of there every day and tried to be funny and available and still a proper father to my kids. I went out to dinner, played tennis and went fishing even though I secretly felt like dying. It made me wretch but I doubled my calories to avoid wasting away; I shopped for nice looking clothes, got up, dressed my best, walked the kids to school and chatted with the parents every day. I refused to lay in the dark even though I often wanted and needed to and I quickly discovered it was working for me. Sometimes just behaving normally, even if you fake it, can make you feel normal and on good days, it can actually make you be normal. I strongly recommend to cancer patients to live fully during treatment as much as you are able. You don't need to be defined by your disease and you should find small ways to take back your life by living it.

*From the mouths of babes (and their moms)*

When I took the kids to school every day, the younger ones on the playground would just horrify their moms with indelicate questions. "What's wrong with you? Why are you bald? Are you going to die like my grandma did?" Kids say whatever they are thinking and I've never met a cancer patient who wasn't refreshed by it. Even very young children understand much more than we give them credit for and having been around young cancer kids, they confide that they know more about their prognosis than their parents think they do. Parents always underestimate what kids can handle. "I have cancer, it's a disease spreading around my body and I'm trying to beat it before it beats me." They never look at me funny again; kids are quick to accept hard things.

Boys and girls are different. At least mine are. We didn't raise them with gender focus, but Gavin liked trucks, trains and natural disaster books from the very beginning, while Zoe loved animals and stories about fairies and dance. When I got cancer, Gavin was very interested in the mechanics of it all. He wanted to know why it happened, what exactly needed to be done about it, and how it all worked. He was serious and wanted more than kid-friendly answers. Zoe's maternal grandfather had recently died from cancer and she had more emotional concerns and questions. What I didn't know until later was that while they focused on different things, both had extremely deep factual and emotional involvement with my disease and very much understood my prognosis, the risks and what it all could mean. Just 8 and 6 years old, they got it, and were able to cope. They helped take care of me and carried quite a load with grace.  Every family is different but we decided to not hide or sugar coat things. We felt they were too intuitive anyway and it's hard to hide a sick, bald, pale man where their dad used to be. We felt they would be more suspicious and worried if they sensed we weren't forthcoming about it all so we put the cards on the table. For our family it was the right move. It would have been too stressful hiding and I worried it would be too surprising, a breach of trust if I did, in fact, have to die.

At Gavin's school, every kid was assigned to make a speech about something of interest they had done with their family. Most of the kids talked about an exotic family vacation, adopting a dog or something else mundane. Gavin asked me if it would be ok to explain my situation and how the family was working as a team to beat my cancer. I worried that it would be a bit heavy for fifth grade but I didn't want him to feel it was a taboo subject and I sensed he needed to share it. His teacher cried when he told his story with clear eyes, facts and love for his dad—she apparently just lost her father to cancer. She was impressed with his depth of knowledge, emotion but also his solid grounding and readiness to shoulder the burden. Both of my kids get it and they are ok. Team Alcott has never been closer.

*Cancer and modern age social networking*

Parents are more complex than their children are. A bemused

African American friend told me that their well-meaning white friends frequently introduce them to other black people assuming an identity affiliation. It's the same for cancer patients. I can't tell you how many times I've been told about a friend of a friend in Ohio who also has cancer and I should give him a call. "Hi, uh, I'm Susan's other cancer friend, how you doing?" Cancer patients understand that people identify with our struggle, are moved by it, and might even admire our handling of it when they ask us to contact another victim. It's intended as a compliment and it's a way for healthy people to participate in supporting the cancer community. Still, I recommend being selective. Cancer patients can feel defined in other people's eyes by their disease. It feels wrong to us being thrown in with total strangers, just because they also have a disease, and we worry that's all you see.

Bernice disagrees with me on this and rightly points out that many cancer patients seek each other out for help and solicit introductions. There is a Yahoo user group, Twitter and Facebook community for every imaginable subgroup of cancer, with total strangers in constant touch. They are sharing treatment protocols and are offering emotional support and lifelong friendships. They organize charity bike races and get together for social reunions and some seem to use this outlet as their main social anchor, even years after a loved one has died or the cancer has been beaten. There is a large group of cancer-networking enthusiasts who mainly do affiliate because of their shared experience.

I've written already about how empathetic strangers are sometimes best-positioned to offer support and encouragement and these online social networking sites are a perfect sweet spot for that; where else can you gain access to thousands of compatible perfect strangers that you can turn on or off as needed 24-hours per day? There is a downside to this virtual community, however. It can be overwhelming seeing all the human suffering fly-by at broadband speed. Many people in these forums are there for a reason, they have dire circumstances and urgent needs. They are there looking for new ideas and exceptional advice because standard protocols are failing or something is going wrong. My first impression after joining such a group was that there were no good outcomes; I certainly was only hearing about very sad situations. It took awhile to realize that the healthy ones were not there or were just passively lurking. That was me. I started to feel guilty going online and reporting that my scan was still good. "Oh, congratulations!" some would write before getting back to their problem; I could imagine crestfallen faces behind the screens wishing it were them. I hope my positive posts can encourage others.

*Fads, hype and pop-culture consumerism*

Cancer activism is cool now and there are many public displays of belonging to the community. Sometimes you get the feeling that cancer is the latest i-phone. Zazzle.com has an entire "Pink Ribbon Shop" online selling cancer swag...mugs, shoes, and buttons. Tee-shirts, ribbons, and charity walks always get the news vans out to the suburbs, especially with the mayor or congressmen leading the march.

We Americans are good at organizing, merchandising, and branding and it seems to give us comfort throwing those skills at this problem. The motives are all good. Huge amounts of money are raised for charity and so is awareness. Still, this cancer patient can't sometimes help but feel that all the hype risks making cancer over-exposed, dumbed-down, and made to look frivolous. Fads pass and people move on to other earnest concerns quickly. They get issue fatigue. I worry about the "fadding" of cancer.

*Cured or not? Why healthy people need it black or white*

Many people in Cancerville want your cancer to be binary. "But you're cured now, right?" They want to know when it will be done or they might even declare that it already is done after a clean 6-month scan. Very few things are like cancer, stuck in permanent limbo, and it's confusing to people. You get strep throat but then it's done; you break a leg until it's forever healed. People have trouble getting their head around a different model. It is hard to imagine how something so deadly and aggressive can disappear without a trace but come back years later. Few people understand why you need ongoing scans, "Didn't you beat it years ago already?" This is often an uncomfortable situation when you try to explain the nuance of ongoing risk. It's often rebutted, "Yeah, but you've pretty much beat it, right?" There's a strange dance that ensues. You certainly don't want to be a cheerleader winning the debate that it's all still pretty dire so you show some confidence and say something about being cautiously optimistic. Your friend feels social pressure to show faith and confidence in your particular mettle, throws out the caution part, and asserts knowing absolutely that you will beat it. This is proper etiquette and both parties are expected to perform their side of the dance.

*Which floor are you on?*

Just like no one really wants to know when they ask, "How are you doing?" they don't really want to end an encounter with you agreeing that the battle continues and it could still end badly. Cancer patients understand this and it creates stress. We often feel like we jumped out of a tenth-floor window and are congratulated by people on the seventh floor—"see you're still ok!" It's uncomfortable socially to pass by your floor and awkward to mention the sidewalk that is fast approaching (unless the firemen get that safety net out in time). It is less awkward for everyone in Cancerville if we all just agree that a safe landing is coming. So we proceed to next floor and hope for the best.

*The cancer oracle*

When you get cancer, especially during treatment or remission, people expect that you have developed some Yoda-like enlightenment and have something to teach. There is some degree of pressure here as you are expected to perform and produce bonafide inspiration sometimes several times per day. People want to know what you learned and how you used the wake-up call of cancer to throw off the chains of your previous horrible and purposeless life to do something great. Lance and many cancer patients talk about the ironic "gift" of cancer and how it's the best thing that ever happened to them. I refuse to occupy that role so easily. The truth is that cancer is crap and while it has given me some perspective, it's totally not worth it and I'd happily be a little less wise, thank you! I definitely don't get as worked up over small things now but I do get worked up instead over big cancer things and that's a bad trade. There's really nothing at all redeeming about it and I'm sorry that people want there to be a "silver lining". There isn't one.

As for big changes, many people tell me they would drop out and join Green Peace, do something really socially relevant, or travel the world. That's when I ask, "So why are you still working at that insurance company?" I feel it's a shame if you have to get cancer to figure out that you hate your life or have the wrong priorities and values. I never had that impulse. I like my life, my wife, my family and my situation and if I didn't, I would have changed it. If you don't like your life now, trust me, cancer won't help you fix it. Better get on with change now.

For those of you who play cards, cancer is like being dealt four shiny diamonds in a row and it's time to bet with one more card to come. The next card could complete a flush (a full rich life!) or you could be dealt a club and fold with nothing at all. You just get no useful life-planning information when you get cancer. You could die very soon…or not at all. This is hard to plan a career change or a "drop out" scenario around. Alas, most cancer patients end up staying in school, going back to the job, and other boring routine things. Some do get a motorcycle and a girlfriend and grow a ponytail. Better late than never to discover yourself I guess. Most of us still have families to support, bills to pay, insurance to keep. I personally found incredible joy in the routine. You don't appreciate normalcy until it is taken away from you by force in the middle of the night. It is a privilege to work and use your brain and I missed it when it was taken away from me.

Cancer patients need some routine and normalcy in their life and people should stop expecting them to do something more exotic when they get sick. Battling for their life and enduring medieval-style treatment tortures is exotic enough, so please let us find some solace going back to our regular boring lives! Cancer patients are already working on the most meaningful and socially relevant project possible: saving our life. And that, Luke Skywalker, takes a lot of wisdom to understand.

*Inside the head of a patient*

In Chapter 2, I wrote about the feeling of inadequacy taking on cancer and the burden of measuring up to the community's expectation for heroism. But there are darker things running around a newly diagnosed patient's head and some beautiful things too. On the dark side, I felt guilty for what I was doing to my family. It wasn't modern to think this way but suddenly I saw myself as head of household, breadwinner and protector of the homestead and I was angry and feeling guilty for putting them at risk. There was a college fund to earn and young minds to shape into good citizens and wife to companion with into our old age. I would never leave them voluntarily and I was shocked that a tiny bump on my face might force me to abandon them suddenly. I never dreamed I could be such a bad father and husband.

Then envy took over. I saw some other man taking over my life, moving into my house, marrying my wife, throwing a ball with my son, giving my daughter away at her wedding. I could visualize being replaced by a photo on the shelf fading to black every year. I felt weak, scarred and unattractive, a lemon that my family was stuck with. At my darker moments, I thought I should leave them quietly in the night. My wife was still young and beautiful, what if I hung on as a broken, disfigured mess for just enough years to drain her of her beauty and youth? What if I siphoned off the family's nest egg and became scary to my young children as things deteriorated? The kids were young enough to probably forget me if I left immediately but if I hung on and dependency grew, maybe I would scar them permanently. Maybe I should release them from my destiny. No one knew how seriously I considered this.

If your wife or husband is fighting cancer, they might be thinking exactly like I was. They might seem skeptical of your love and testing of your commitment and you can resent that given all you're doing. Maybe you're thinking, "Can't he see I'm standing by him, why does he keep questioning my love?" Or maybe she's detaching, backing away from you and the children, and snapping at you. "Does she want to leave us and have a final adventure?" It might be the contrary. This is a complex emotional time. Behaviors may be motivated by things too dark for others in Cancerville to understand.

Only a scared cancer patient could think of disappearing in the night forever abandoning their young family—and see it as their last loving and most unselfish act. Be careful about what you think you see. It's popular in social sciences today to believe that all human behavior and motivation is selfish. Supposedly, we do nothing but for self-interest; just cynical acts to self-impress or score metaphysical points. I now know this isn't true. When my moment came and I had to face losing it all, the guilt, envy and anger left me.

*The Beatles were right*

A simple clarity unfolds when the reality of cancer hits. I didn't need more life but I knew I had more to give to my family. I would do anything for them including if I had to suffer and lose my dignity and chase tumors until I couldn't anymore. I resolved to do exactly that. I didn't leave in the middle of the night because I had hope. My wife made me still feel wanted and centered in her future plans. Bernice made a point out of long-range planning with me. She took me out to look at houses to buy and renovate together. We talked about doing the work ourselves and about starting a business together. I got the message. I was still "Plan A" and we had a future together. My kids still needed me too and showed me every day how centered I was in their life plan. They wanted me to teach them to ski next winter; Gavin hoped I could get him ready to be a pitcher next spring. Zoe asked one day if it would be ok to still live in the house with mom and me after she got married and became a vet. I love little girls! There was still a lot to give.

I don't buy into trendy social science academics. Everything isn't selfish; it isn't a one sided "take" equation that guides and motivates our lives. I prefer the wisdom of the Beatles who famously wrote: "And in the end, the love you take is equal to the love you make."

*A normal day in Cancerville*

I always looked forward to my friend, Rob, calling when I was sick. Rob didn't change at all. He called about as often as before and would tell me about the crappy Stones concert he just saw in Chicago or about neighborhood gossip, his job and world politics. We'd chat, laugh and never mention the elephant in the room. For Rob, I was still Scott and not "Cancer-Scott". He was keeping up with my situation through other channels but didn't let it become the basis of our relationship. It was same with my friend from work, Jacques. I was no longer his boss, I had no power, but he called me every week at the same time to get advice, talk about business, and share with me news from the water cooler. It meant a lot to still be needed and it kept me engaged, sharp, and feeling relevant. Every cancer patients needs at least one Rob or Jacques. If you live in Cancerville, U.S.A, every once in awhile, just act normally so we can too.

# 6

## The Blame Game

Lance writes about negotiating with cancer: "If the deal is that I never cycle again, but I get to live, I'll take it." Maybe it was the cycling that did it to him after all. How many of you figured he did it to himself sitting cramped on that painful tiny seat for years?

This kind of thinking isn't just reserved for celebrities. When you get cancer, you soon find out that many people around you think it's your fault and they are driven to find the reason and assign blame. There are different reasons for this but it is nearly universal and often the patient himself participates in this blame game. I believe healthy people hate the idea that they are not in control. They want to confirm that you either did something wrong or failed to sufficiently do something good that they believe in. This way, healthy people can go on in the comfort that they won't get cancer because…

Others want to assign blame so that the cause can be quarantined—a very common impulse of the patient himself. Often this leads to conspiracy theories with anecdotal "clusters" being identified around variously questioned water supplies, cellular phone towers, radon gas zones, overhead electric wires, and up-river industrial parks.

There's good reason for this general blame impulse. We have all been taught by news reports, popular books and public health advocates that cancer is caused by bad behavior. Some of this is hard to refute. We all know the clear relation between tobacco, sun exposure, asbestos, toxic dumps and cancer. But from there, if you want to assign blame, there's something for everybody. Eventually you will be told how you failed to save your soul by the Church of Green Tea Adherents, the stress-busting meditation enthusiasts, the anti-red meat lobby, the anti-industrial ecologists and the proponents of the "red wine miracle." Good friends from all faiths will tell you it's proven that being active in their place of worship statistically lowers the incidence of cancer and other illnesses. Others are smugly satisfied that their vitamin supplements, their low-impact parabolic exercise machine, their new age holistic doctor or their annual $2,000 Total Health Check™ will protect them from their own genetics and the cold harsh laws of probability. Some may even try to dissuade you from traditional medical interventions after you get cancer. They argue against chemotherapy in favor of various eastern herbal treatments or unregulated supplements that have been "proven" to cure cancer. In the whispered hush of conspiracy theorists, you're told that the evil corporate agenda is cynically keeping these cures from the masses to prolong the economic cancer bonanza that is western medicine; or sometimes it's the government bureaucracy that is just too slow to approve the "cure" but it's coming in 2015 (and now available in Mexico or China).

As you can imagine, this all gets pretty disheartening for the cancer patient. The guilt sets in quickly. Did I put my life and family at risk by going to McDonald's too often as a teenager? Did I indulge myself on that Starbucks caffeine rush instead of taking that all-healing green tea? Did I climb that stressful ladder of success too much instead of honing my inner peace? Maybe I drank too much in college or failed to go to the gym enough or I forgot the vitamin too many mornings. The possibilities for how you failed yourself and your family are endless. And if you're the parent of a child with cancer, the guilt and anxiety is even worse. Is it my genes that did it? Did we buy a house in dangerous cancer environment? We should have bought organic!

I think it's hard to argue against precaution. Any reasonable person would agree with taking care of yourself and avoiding high-risk behavior as a hedge against cancer and other diseases. Unfortunately, the opposite is not true. Too many people are unreasonable zealots believing that your problem was 100% preventable by following the dogma of their preferred solution.

When you get cancer, you need to develop a thick skin and anticipate the question. I was surprised how many people asked me flat out, "What did you do to yourself to get it?" I was surprised how many times I was scolded for not being a vegan or for living on the east coast, or for working too hard or not working out hard enough. I'm sure everyone meant well. But I couldn't help but feel many people just wanted to reassure themselves that they couldn't be me. After all, I'm scary to many people. I didn't smoke, chew tobacco or do anything else extreme or obviously wrong. I wasn't obese, sedentary, unduly stressed or in a high-risk group. There was no cancer in my family and we lived in upscale and clean environments. In fact, the cancer I got seems to follow no pattern at all other than it affects otherwise healthy and usually very young people. This is the case more often than I ever knew. Lung cancer does hit non-smokers. Zen-master vegans like Steve Jobs from Apple, Inc. get pancreatic cancer for no apparent reason. There are entire hospitals dedicated to childhood cancers and brain tumors that have no particular cause, affecting young and old, fit and fat and sometimes world-class athletes.   Like a bug that shows up in computer software, sometimes the human software just screws up in a single cell out of a trillion, an accident in synchronization, a mistake in cell fusion, a flaw in the tumor-suppressing gene of that particular cell. Lightning does strike. With all of our cells and complexity, it's a miracle it doesn't happen to everyone; still, about 40% of us will get cancer some time in our life.[6]

My own experience has made me more fatalistic about life and the folly of believing that we are in control. I think it's a very American mentality to believe we can steer, fix, and control things—we're high performing people that made it to the moon and it's in our psyche to believe everything is in our power. There's a television ad offering a cure for every malady. Cholesterol, allergies, erectile dysfunction, and restless leg syndrome can all be cured with a pill. Gym memberships, magic herbs, the Life Extension Institute, hormone replacement therapy, organic foods and an aisle of vitamins and supplements at the grocery store all promise they can make a difference and help us beat the odds. I'm not so sure. I watched bald 8-year-old boys from all around the world in the chemo rooms. They didn't smoke or have job stress or years of bad behaviors. And I saw their sometimes-overweight doctors, nurses and therapists huddled outside the same hospital having a smoke or scarfing down a hot dog all apparently in better condition than the people in their care. There's no justice in cancer.

I know what you're thinking. That's all anecdotal. I can beat the curve. I will be spared. I do the right things and avoid the wrong things and it's proven it's going to matter statistically. Are you so sure that it matters—that you can control your own mortality and behave your way around the risk probability? Take a look at the Social Security Administration's Actuarial Life Table (see Table 1).

What this table shows is amazing. Life expectancy at birth is 77 years. By age sixty, nearly 90% of us are still kicking including all the car accidents, hurricane and war deaths, gang-bang drive-by shootings, drug overdoses, poverty, malnutrition, AIDS, suicides, murders and infant mortality (which accounts for most of the death by 60). The 90% who make it includes obese people, chain smokers, beef jerky eaters, supplement takers, stress buckets and their vegan, Olympian marathon-running, Zen-master counterparts; they are all in the data. They've all made it safely to 80% of their life expectancy. It is statistically stunning that in spite of huge behavioral variance humans are so robust. And then it suddenly happens. Bam! 25% of us are gone by the next 10 years and 35% go five years after that. Then it falls off the cliff completely. It's like clockwork. We expire in large swaths at our expiration date across virtually all nutritional and behavioral subgroups.

I'm no statistician but the fact that there is such huge standard error in behavior co-existing with robust survival rates across that standard error—well I think it means green tea can't be *that* magical. Even a layman can tell that what mainly kills people is age (and being male apparently!) no matter what you do.

I'm not saying all the anti-oxidant potions, Lipitor, magic herbs, megadose vitamins, low glycemic index diets, exercise strategies and risk avoidance is pointless. No reasonable person would argue that. Quality of life and peace of mind also matters and is greatly affected by the behavior choices we make. And maybe the bad boys are more often in the rare "early death" statistics; maybe they are first in line when we all start dropping in our seventies a few years ahead of the best behaving; maybe the yogurt eaters really are the lucky few who live to be 100. I'm not so sure. Look around, everyone is obese, sedentary, stressed, over caffeinated and/or sleep deprived or has some other deficit; so exactly who are these masses making it to life expectancy? It can't be just the tea drinkers!

After my cancer, I've accepted that I'm really not in control. I've stopped the guilt and doubt about what I did or didn't do. I respect the fate and destiny revealed by the Actuarial Life Table. I have

Table 1:     **Period Life Table, 2005**[7]

| Age Now | Male | | | Female | | |
|---|---|---|---|---|---|---|
| | Death Rate | # Alive at Age | Life Exp. | Death Rate | # Alive at Age | Life Exp. |
| 0 | 0.007566 | 100,000 | 74.81 | 0.006156 | 100,000 | 79.95 |
| 1 | 0.000522 | 99,243 | 74.38 | 0.000416 | 99,384 | 79.45 |
| 2 | 0.000358 | 99,192 | 73.42 | 0.000257 | 99,343 | 78.48 |
| 3 | 0.000255 | 99,156 | 72.45 | 0.000181 | 99,318 | 77.5 |
| 4 | 0.000204 | 99,131 | 71.47 | 0.000155 | 99,300 | 76.52 |
| 60 | 0.011908 | 84,891 | 20.42 | 0.007365 | 91,036 | 23.53 |
| 65 | 0.017609 | 79,061 | 16.73 | 0.011366 | 87,051 | 19.49 |
| 70 | 0.027295 | 71,108 | 13.3 | 0.01816 | 81,235 | 15.69 |
| 75 | 0.042921 | 60,102 | 10.26 | 0.029029 | 72,612 | 12.24 |
| 80 | 0.068216 | 45,986 | 7.62 | 0.047669 | 60,540 | 9.16 |
| 85 | 0.111834 | 29,666 | 5.41 | 0.082854 | 44,411 | 6.54 |
| 86 | 0.123673 | 26,349 | 5.03 | 0.092709 | 40,731 | 6.08 |
| 87 | 0.136793 | 23,090 | 4.67 | 0.103657 | 36,955 | 5.65 |
| 88 | 0.151241 | 19,931 | 4.34 | 0.115742 | 33,124 | 5.25 |
| 89 | 0.167026 | 16,917 | 4.02 | 0.128995 | 29,291 | 4.87 |
| 90 | 0.18414 | 14,091 | 3.72 | 0.143437 | 25,512 | 4.52 |
| 91 | 0.202559 | 11,497 | 3.45 | 0.159077 | 21,853 | 4.19 |
| 92 | 0.222243 | 9,168 | 3.2 | 0.175914 | 18,377 | 3.89 |
| 93 | 0.243144 | 7,130 | 2.97 | 0.193937 | 15,144 | 3.61 |
| 94 | 0.265201 | 5,397 | 2.77 | 0.213123 | 12,207 | 3.36 |
| 95 | 0.287099 | 3,965 | 2.59 | 0.232548 | 9,605 | 3.13 |

come to accept that sometimes lightning does just strike. If I die from this disease before age 60, it's a statistical fluke that almost never happens, even to those with the worst behaviors, which certainly isn't me! If it happens to me, I guess it's my fate. A religious person might think of it as God's will; a statistician might see it as a random probability occurrence; a geneticist might see Darwinian forces at work. In any case, it is clearly bad luck and bad luck can happen to the best and worst behaving of us all. Even Lance Armstrong can get cancer. Like the turn of a card, someone has to be in the statistical noise. Why shouldn't it be me…or you?

It's taken two years but I've stopped blaming myself now. I hope others can too.

# 7

# "Scanxiety"

Second-round chemotherapy all but killed me. My veins had collapsed and it took many tries to get any needle into me. I had bruises up and down my arms from failed attempts and by this time, my muscle tissue, bone mass and heart were pretty much eaten away. My brain no longer worked the way it used to. I had trouble helping my second-grader do single-digit math computation; I seemed to have lost "muscle memory" and processing speed. I was unable to keep track of the continuity of things that happened in the past and had no recall of certain visits and events. I was also subject to sensory overload. I couldn't manage a room with more than two people; it was difficult to follow the conversation and process all that was going on.

On the other hand, like a savant that compensates a deficit, I found I was processing complex information better than ever and was functioning mentally at a very high level. I was writing strategic papers for my office that stunned my bosses and motivated significant strategic moves. I started reading physics books by the shopping cart and learned about equations behind Einstein's relativity theories. This re-arranging of the brain is called simply "Chemo-Brain" which seems refreshingly straight for a medical term.

And suddenly, it was done. The last set of injections was complete. All that remained was to partially die again over three weeks to let the last session work its poisonous magic. Miraculously, I did this evil round all outpatient. I never missed a round, never went into toxic shock, never crashed with a fever, never succumbed to infection and never spent a single night in the hospital. I handled the convulsions, pain, and shock of it all and made it through.

When I got home, Bernice had a cake ready with an over-the-top picture made out of icing. Small circles were scattered around the cake with a line striking though it, "No Small Round Blue Cells" it said with an exclamation point, referring to my cancer. Bernice understood before I did that it was important to mark these events and progress points. The same thinking behind the radiation chart, Bernice wanted me to see that I was succeeding and putting things behind me. It's a great mental trick and I recommend all patients set up milestones and celebrate achievements.

When Lance finished his treatment, he got back on the bike and like most cancer patients, after a few false starts, Lance eventually went back to his life and work. He was ambivalent at first and recognized that he needed to heal his mind and soul after his body. After a failed attempt at retiring and bumming around, Lance literally got back on the bike. He focused on training, getting married, having a baby and becoming a global celebrity and world champion. If Lance ever looked back after his "all clear", you can't find it in his book. Champions know when they have won the game. He speaks in the past tense about cancer and how he beat it in interviews and television commercials all over the world. It wasn't that way for me. After finishing my treatment, I found it increasingly difficult and carried around a chronic, low-grade depression. I had moved from active treatment to checking if it had worked. "Scans" refer to the battery of CT, MRI and PET scans that are done at regular intervals after treatment is done to see if you are still cancer free. It's kind of like getting a report card every 90 days except this report card tells you if all you did was a waste of time and if you are going to die or not.

I think there is a bit of post-traumatic stress that comes when all the crisis activity stops. It's surreal when they tell you, "It's done, go now." Just like that. You finally get a moment to reflect on what has happened to you. You leave the hospitals and active care and there's no ceremony, no graduation ritual, no blue ribbon. I feel like I can approximate the feeling of war veterans taken overnight out of combat and dropped back into society blind to the trauma they experienced.

Even though the punishing treatment of chemo and radiation is over, the mental anguish not only persists, it actually amplifies. That's because treatment is a physical but also mental security blanket. You're being cared for, given medicine—you are carpet-bombing the cancer and getting an incredible amount of oversight and personal attention. When it's done, the training wheels are off and you are without defenses just waiting and hoping that it doesn't come back.

Understand that when treatment is over, you've done all you can do. The doctors keep no reserve. Maximum dosages and full guns are unloaded during treatment and every bullet has already been shot. If the cancer returns after that, it's very disheartening. It means the treatment available just doesn't work and there are not a lot of good options. A recurrence means more surgery, if it's operable, or maybe a clinical trial with new chemotherapy experiments. After a bike ride through the woods to clear my head, I sat down and wrote a poem in one pass that still best captures my mindset during this stressful time:

## "Borrowed Time"

Deathly ill but feeling fine, hard to wrap around my mind, Am I well? The
next scan will tell if I'm living on borrowed time.
Am I living on borrowed time?

"Chin up, man you'll make it through, Lance won his battle, so can you. Keep
the proper attitude, you're gonna make it too!"
Another platitude.

Endless tests and activity, obscuring grim reality, just a coping strategy, for
filling up my time.
Are they messing with my mind?

Can I trust what they do or say, or is it just the only way, to make me go home
today, feeling more sublime?
Am I dying in my prime?

It's all become the new routine, needles, pills and toxic screens, this bald man
where I used to be, forever burned in family scenes.
Do they still remember me?

Treatment done I did the time, back to work and the daily grind, need to leave
this hell behind, and capture my old self.
If I can just keep up my health.

Six months now I'm on parole, the chemo took a heavy toll, I'm free for now
but can't escape the crime.
It's lurking all the time.

Am I well or just okay? The "rock-star" doctors just can't say, I mark another
living day and search for peace of mind.
It's very hard to find.

It's never very far away, just another ninety days. Am I well? The next scan
will tell if I'm living on borrowed time.
Am I living on borrowed time?

It's a humbling experience watching what you can do to yourself psychologically during this time. Cancer patients refer to this as "scanxiety". I'm not an especially hysterical person but when I was released, I became a certifiable hypochondriac. Right before my regular 90-day follow-up scans, I would usually find a lump somewhere; feel a pain, experience eye twitches and headaches. You name it. Most of this would go away immediately after the scans revealed no problems to worry about. Even after becoming aware of this pattern, I was unable to stop developing symptoms immediately before scans. Scanxiety is complicated by actual treatment-related side effects that appear over time and show up in routine scans (see Chapter 12 to understand "late effects" from cancer treatment). It turns out that I did have swollen nodes, nerve damage and numbness from my treatment and I was feeling real, not imaginary, things. Before cancer, you probably always experienced tingles, twinges and pain and didn't think a thing about it. After cancer, you track it all and are on red alert.

*Head fakes and winks*

Waiting for the results of follow-up scans is the highest trauma you can experience. Cancer patients can get paranoid and read into things that aren't there. And sometimes there's a week or more after getting a scan and having the results read out by your doctor. To handicap that, I found I was trying to read the tone in the room while the scan was being done. Why was the technician so cold and quick to get me out, does she know the scan had a problem? That scan took a lot more time, were they going back and forth over a problem area? Sometimes my doctor called with good results right away instead of making me wait for the office visit; other times he was silent and I assumed he was making me come in rather than give bad news on the phone. I'd rush to answer every call. One time after a scan, the doctor ordered a blood test—did the scan flag something that he needed blood to confirm? In all of the above cases, it was plain paranoia. Doctors are busy, they travel. Sometimes they call. Sometimes they think to do a blood test. Sometimes the scans go longer. There's no reason. All you can do is wait and hope for good news.

And that's what we mainly do. Wait. And we constantly re-live that "open door moment" that got us here in the first place. Oncologists are always late to the open door moment, sometimes hours late. You wait in the lobby like a child outside of the principal's office hoping to avoid detention. Eventually reception calls you and moves you to a sterile private room which means the doctor is getting closer to reading out your verdict. He probably hasn't even read your scan reports yet and is doing it just before bursting in. You wait, while he deliberates over your life. Then there's a knock, the door opens, and if it's good news, there is no small talk. A happy face, big smile, and a thumbs-up enter the room, "Don't worry, it's all fine!" Your blood pressure falls and you make nice small talk. He tells you that you look great and you tell him you feel great.

Typically, this is when the "by the way" remark comes. When you are checked for cancer recurrence with CT scans, MRIs and PET scans, they see everything going on in your body. Anyone you put through such a battery of tests will show something but it's especially true for people who have had trauma, surgery, caustic poison and high-energy radiation blowing through their cells. The tests show inflammation, swelling, elevated metabolic activities as well as nodules, scuffs and lesions. "By the way, your thyroid gland reads a little hot in the PET scan but I'm not worried about it, probably just radiation effect, I'll order an ultrasound next month just to confirm." And just like that, your moment of elation is popped and you go back on the worry wagon. After almost every scan, something inconclusive like that showed up—always probably nothing to worry about. So naturally, I did worry. It's rare that you get a passing grade without footnotes. And this keeps the stress level high. Intellectually you develop expectations and tell yourself you've been through it before, but emotionally it's still very hard. Usually this is about the time an acquaintance insists, "You're cured though, right?"

Because we can imagine things and dream up symptoms, I recommend new cancer patients take good digital photos of their body and write down pains and sensations they feel. This is very helpful later when you think that area near the surgery might have changed a little and you start talking yourself into worrying about it. Photos usually prove me wrong, "No, that was always there." For me, I was able to worry less about the latest sensation when my record book of other things all variously proved to be nothing. It's a good toolkit for controlling imagination. I also remind patients on a 90-day scan cycle that on average, a recurrence might be 45 days old by the time of your next scan and it's very unlikely that you would actually feel anything that young…so yes, you probably are imagining it. This has gotten me through difficult periods.

The scan procedure is no picnic either. For a CT scan, you drink a liter of a sweet Crystal Light contrast solution on an empty stomach; it's cold, swells your belly, and makes you need to urinate. But you have to sit perfectly still in the machine for up to a half hour. Midway through the procedure, a nurse injects you with an iodine solution which for many people is incredibly nauseating. You can feel it hit your veins and its spreads a sickening warm sensation through every part of your body. At some point, it cumulates and you fight with all of your will to not throw up; you can picture the liter of red Crystal Light projected over the million-dollar CT machine and you try to hold on. For me, the sensation lasts 50 seconds; I know because there is a digital counter on the machine and I've learned I just need to hold on for that long before the nausea passes. It's truly a miserable experience.

The PET scan is worse. You have to fast all night and load up on Crystal Light, but this time they also inject a radioactive isotope into your veins. The CT scan is looking for tumors and takes a million static photos of slices of your body. The PET scan is looking for biological activity associated with cancer and it outputs full motion animation of your body. It's looking to see if cancer cells munch away on the injected isotope and with this clever trick, they can tell where a tumor will develop even before the cells have gathered themselves into a visible tumor. The PET takes about an hour and you're struggling to remain still while needing to pee. When you leave, you get an airport security card because the isotope in your veins can trigger homeland security checks—apparently, after a PET scan, you read like a dirty-nuke device.

If you are supporting a cancer patient, the first two years after treatment are the hardest. Lance doesn't write much about it but I guarantee even he had significant fear, uncertainty and doubt during this period of his recovery. Everyone wants to move on and most do the minute your treatment is over. You are declared "ok" (at least for the moment) and that's good enough for most people. Back to normal! And it's easy to start forgetting. The hair is back and the sickly pallor is gone. Things seem like they were. But it's still living in the patient's head and he knows he has less support now to talk about it. Patients at this stage are more alone than they've ever been and are often covering. Look after your loved ones especially during this time.

Lance's celebrity exploded after cancer and he became a world spokesman with accolades and trophies and a saint-like status. The rest of us just go back to work with a heavy burden in the background. It surprised me to conquer the first rounds of this battle and find myself back on the mat like this later; still fearful and doubtful about my chances. Lance expects to win hard races. I was surprised to still be alive. Was I living on borrowed time?

# 8

## Cancer, Inc.

When I look back on all I did: surgery, chemo, radiation, and more chemo, I'm struck by the impressive feat of cancer management. Fighting cancer is like planning and fighting a war; it's an enormous logistical and operational challenge and it has to be executed flawlessly while bombs are falling all around you. Your partner in this war is Cancer Inc., the complex bureaucracy of doctors, medical personnel, and staff involved with fighting your cancer. You learn quickly that not all teams are the same and even the best ones have peculiar processes and cultures that sometimes break down if not handled with care.

If you're new to the cancer community and still have the luxury of choosing the organization that will treat you, there are some critical things to consider first. If you're in active treatment already, in remission or battling a late recurrence, a deeper understanding of the organization, personalities, and processes behind your treatment can help you get the most out of Cancer, Inc.

In Lance's book, you get a glance at some of the people involved with his treatment but less insight is given about the organization that works (and sometimes doesn't work) behind the individuals. I think it's important to understand who you will be dealing with, what they're like, how they think and the inter-workings between them.

*Your primary care physician*

Remember this person? Very often, you entered Lance's club because your primary care physician, Ob-Gyn, or family doctor ordered a scan or a biopsy for some initial complaint. She may be a long-time family friend and someone in your community whom you trust and are comfortable with. Cancer patients may struggle with how to integrate this doctor into ongoing cancer management and it gets harder for long- term patients to figure out the proper placement of this role.

During the initial blur of a cancer diagnosis, this doctor will largely be left behind, especially during active cancer care. That's because even basic things like rashes, colds, infections, and fevers need to be analyzed and treated within the context of cancer management. There are no longer routine medical issues when you get cancer. If something comes up, the oncologist has to know and has to be the captain for dealing with it. A sore throat might be a recurrence or a treatment side effect, or if just an infection, it could be a threat during chemotherapy. Nothing is an isolated incident when you have cancer.

Some patients try to insert their family physician (or Uncle Jim the doctor) into Cancer, Inc. during active cancer treatment and it can be an unnatural construction. It can create friction, bruise egos and confuse the bureaucracy about who "owns you" and where accountability/responsibility for you ultimately sits. Cancer patients need to be very careful to not divide ownership and accountability or decisions can be delayed, communications can be fractured, and the machine can break down.

If you want an "outside" player to participate in your cancer management, you need to be sure that Cancer, Inc. is comfortable with that conceptually and operationally. Should the results of your scans and blood tests be sent to your uncle G.P. for him to discuss with you instead of the oncologist leading that? If you complicate flows like that, beware later of finger pointing and frequent communications breakdowns. Extra layers fragment the project and things can fall through the cracks with too many hand-offs. My strong recommendation is to limit outside interference during active cancer treatment; choose a captain that has the accountability and authority to manage your cancer and all your medical needs during active treatment.

The role of a primary care doctor will re-emerge later when active treatment stops, especially during long periods of remission. You can't bother your cancer doctor for every flu and routine medical need so your primary care doctor becomes the lead again during this stage of cancer management. It's important that this primary doctor knows your history, is well versed and alert to signs of cancer recurrence and late-effect problems that can come from earlier cancer treatment (see Chapter 12). There's a nice balance in this arrangement: during early days, your cancer doctor takes over many G.P. functions but later during remission, your G.P. needs to raise his cancer monitoring skills. Over time, it evens out!

*Your oncologist*

The job of an oncologist is to be the captain of your ongoing treatment plan. He commands a team of people to figure out what disease you have and then designs and oversees that team to implement the treatment plan. What's interesting is the team that he drives does not entirely work for him hierarchically and some on the team may even see themselves as superior or at least peers. This can cause some organizational side-effects that I'll get into later. Since the oncologist takes over much of the primary care role, many patients want this cancer doctor to have qualities and style reminiscent of the family doctor—patients are often disappointed and confused if they don't. But your oncologist has many roles and needs to be many things. He is not your family doctor. You may have better and more productive interactions with him if you understand his role and mindset differently.

*Inside the mind of the oncologist*

There is no other profession with so many brilliant, high-powered, supremely credentialed and committed people, all failing constantly. It's hard being a cancer doctor. Most are very high achievers but spend much of their day overseeing bad outcomes. They are scientists, trained and oriented to be thinking about microscopic cells, but in practice, they find much of their life is about comforting and reassuring people. Many doctors in the field are wrongly matched for the reality of the patient side of their job. Most patients want a nice cancer doctor with good "soft skills"; one who will comfort, nurture and give assurances. The reality is the best doctors didn't get into the field because they were gifted in soft skills. Some of the best may not be that nice at all but have many other critical skills.

Oncologists are strategists. No two cancer situations are the same and your oncologist and his team need to "call an audible" when your case file hits their desk. Standard protocol called for concurrent radiation and chemotherapy for my cancer, which normally appears in the arms and legs. That can't work for a tumor in the more sensitive head and neck area so they planned a different sequence. Some patient-specific decisions like that are needed for virtually every case of cancer.

Cancer treatment is a chess game that unfolds based on previous moves and how you react to ongoing treatments. The team will adjust doses, frequency and even throw a "Hail Mary" pass if all else fails. In cancer management, the playbook often is thrown out the window. A good reassuring guy is wonderful during that chess game but it's critical that your oncologist has a team, a process and acumen for quarterbacking his way through the ups and downs of your game. It is an active and "tough call" business and your oncologist must be a steely field marshal at the right moments. In some cases, it might even be preferable if he's not too much your friend and emotionally involved. It can be hard to send your friend into a crushing radioactive storm that will cause collateral damage, even if it's necessary.

Oncologists are also large team leaders, much more so than your family doctor. A strong oncologist can attract a great team, get favors done and can use his status in Cancer, Inc. to get you the best surgeon (who on paper is booked until next year). If he needs it and has the gravitas, pathology might get done a bit quicker for him if he picks up the phone, and a scan can be squeezed in and analyzed same day if you're stressing. The oncologist is an operational leader and the good ones have designed a patient process and hired administrative leaders, attracted the best interns onto his analysis/treatment design team and he runs a tight office that answers your calls, gets you reports and makes the considerable administration burden light. Day to day, he is more of a COO than he is Marcus Welby.

Many oncologists at bigger hospitals have a double life. They are doing drug development, clinical trials, and research while writing, teaching, and making rounds at the hospital. They may sit on boards or have outside work for drug companies. Some are literally medical rock-stars catering to the stars and chairing black tie affairs at charity auctions. Often on just one day a week, they pay their bills and see up to twenty patients for office visits and follow-ups. It's that day that they need to be patient, accessible and caring human beings and it's hard to go from molecular scientist to counselor on six hours sleep. Amazingly, some oncologists master the skill of being both. I was very fortunate to have a leader in his field that also turned out to be one of the most caring, sincere and open human beings I've ever met. It's very rare to find one person so developed in both areas.

When thinking about your oncologist and your expectations of him, consider all the roles he must play and all the skills he must have. Accept the possibility that a small deficit in soft skills can be offset by his other attributes and be thankful if you're lucky enough to get both!

*The surgeon*

Unfortunately, surgery is all too common with cancer and often it's needed again years later because of recurrences. The surgeon is one member of the team that could have limited soft skills. It takes a certain kind of person to slice you open and hold steady around your carotid artery while the iPod sets some mood music in the operating room! The surgeon is a ninja and not a counselor. To borrow a business metaphor, your oncologist is the "account manager" (you are the account) but the surgeon is the factory. Any buyer knows that the account manager is important but he can't make up for bad products and a bad factory. Unfortunately, many patients never look beyond the oncologist. Most cancers require surgery and this may be the most important procedure you will get. The strategy, skill and execution of that surgeon are often the most determining factors in whether you live or die.

Often, patients shop for the oncologist but take the assigned surgeon, no questions asked. This is a mistake. Top oncologists often can secure a top surgeon as part of his oversight of your overall treatment plan but you should know who is doing the cutting and you need to participate in his strategic approach. I gave the surgeon a green light to do radical surgery if he felt it would improve my chances. Without that guidance, he might have a made a compromise on my behalf assuming I would prefer to avoid too much disfigurement. That wasn't my strategy and I wanted it clear.

Surgery is not a standard off-the-shelf procedure and surgical facilities don't all have the same capabilities and services available. A surgeon needs to assess the situation live and think about creative incisions to remove wide margins without unnecessary destruction of organs, nerves and tissues. It's an on-the-fly, talent-driven skill. A good surgical ward has real time pathology happening during surgery so the surgeon can remove cancer cells without guessing or relying on visual inspection. A good surgeon will excise the tumor "en masse" when possible instead of dividing it into manageable sections first—this avoids leakage and incidental spreading of microscopic cancer cells— which can greatly worsen your prognosis. Proper technique matters and so do capabilities of the surgical ward; you should understand both before the cutting starts.

Cancer surgeons are often the real "rock stars" at Cancer, Inc., and they may not like being interviewed. Still, you should see him before the standard planning and "pre-op" meetings to assess him— even if he came with high recommendations from your oncologist. Has he done a high volume of similar procedures? Can he describe his strategy for getting wide margins while preserving function? Is he listening to your wishes and priorities or does he seem closed to his own way of thinking? Your oncologist may want to manage this interaction gently to avoid bruising egos. Unfortunately, political care is important in Cancer, Inc. like it is with any other organization. Still, once you're knocked out on his operating table, the surgeon has total control; it's better to align before the cutting to avoid waking up surprised. I was lucky again to have a great, patient-centered surgeon.

*Office manager (gatekeeper, scheduler, "SPOC")*

Cancer is an enormous administrative burden. There are hundreds of appointments and procedures that need to be planned, sequenced and followed-up in the right order and paperwork needs to be exchanged between you and many other departments at Cancer, Inc. Good oncologists consider the office manager a vital part of his permanent medical team and he does not rely on college kids, temps or see this as purely incidental administrative activity. More like a paralegal in a law firm than a secretary, the medical office manager has cancer management skills. They need to know that medical intervals are needed between procedures before scheduling them; they need to know how long it takes to get results back from a biopsy or blood work before scheduling downstream procedures. More importantly, they need to know everything about your status and treatment protocol as a medical team member. "Mr. Alcott, you're scheduled for a CT and a PET but I know we usually do a separate head and neck scan, let me check with the doctor if he intended to change that." This kind of intervention is what makes the office manager a critical member of the team.

This person is also a gatekeeper and Single Point of Contact ("SPOC"). Get on the wrong side of the gatekeeper and you may find access to the doctor restricted or appointments less flexible. If you treat the manager as the crucial team member they are, all kinds of things can happen and be brokered at Cancer, Inc. by this magician of logistics. Beware of an oncologist that does not invest in this role. Often a detached, purely administrative, low-level office manager is a sign that your oncologist wants to control access. When this role is reduced to a rotating cast and an answering service, you are cut off and only able to see the doctor on his terms at scheduled office visits (or in an emergency). A connected office manager can listen to your problem and catch the doctor in between patients and let you know what he says. You want to use this role selectively to keep relations good.

When you start with an oncologist, it's critical to ask about his office management process. Inquire if he has an office manager or medical nurse and how you can expect to interact with them. Trust me, during your battle, things will go wrong, symptoms will pop up, fear and questions will hit you. You will want the security of being in touch with someone when that happens and you don't want to feel like you called the switchboard at some faceless Cancer, Inc. I cannot overstate the importance of this role for your survival and recovery. I used this "SPOC" several times during my battle and got helped during emergencies, both real and imagined ones!

*The medical nurse, intern or physician's assistant*

Because your oncologist has many jobs and is rarely sitting at his desk able to speak to you, many oncology teams include a junior medical professional who may be doing his residency or is a professional medical nurse. Often this is the first line that reacts when you get a fever or a reaction to chemo or some unexpected medical development. If you don't get that warm fuzzy feeling from your oncologist but think he might be a great operational and strategic leader, give consideration to this important team member. This person is usually more accessible, more of a people person, less pressed for time and available to you. Their profile is usually younger (interns, medical residents) and nurturing. Many became professional nurses with an eye to the patient management side (rather than the drug development or research side). Often this person can be an alter ego to the oncologist and it can be the best situation to have both. A key theme is to consider the entire team when evaluating your care provider as it can work wonderfully as a system (or not).

*Other important team members*

On the front lines of your battle, you will spend many hours with shift-based chemotherapy nurses, radiation therapy and diagnostic scan technicians, blood/vital sign takers and business office personnel (insurance and payment management). Behind the scenes, you have lab technicians, pathologists and others who supply data and information to the front-line team.

As you can imagine, it's an enormous task managing all the stakeholders and process of cancer treatment. I often felt I needed a personal "project manager" to handle it all; remember you're in no condition physically or mentally to manage the minutia. Typically, a loved one, who is also dealing emotionally with your cancer, has to carry the burden. That same person is also managing the house, the kids, going to work and fighting with the insurance company about bills due. This takes an enormous toll on the entire family and it's why it is critical to pick a cancer team that operates efficiently and effectively so you can focus on getting better instead of the cancer management process. You have enough to do to survive cancer and you should avoid taking on an unpaid job at Cancer, Inc.

If you are a doctor or medical professional reading this, I'd like to influence you to give new patients an orientation session and booklet. Your team and process should be introduced and not assumed to be obvious to the patient and your way of working should be specified. For patients reading this, I strongly encourage you to ask about the team and their work process before getting started. If you're already in active treatment and things aren't working smoothly, speak up and remember that your oncologist is not just a doctor, he's a team leader and in command of Cancer, Inc.; don't be afraid to ask him to make adjustments to ease operational burdens on you.

*Doctor Shopping*

Newly diagnosed patients have much to consider before picking a team to save their life. But patients in active treatment also frequently need to revisit their treatment choices. Unfortunately, some cancers recur or fail to respond to first-line treatments driving patients to search for specialty centers with different doctors, clinical trials and novel therapies. Too often, cancer patients are out there evaluating another Cancer, Inc. and often under urgent circumstances.

Lance writes extensively about his "doctor shopping" experience literally crossing the country to find the right team to handle his cancer. Not surprisingly, Lance gravitated towards "can do" doctors who were on the cutting edge aspiring to totally defeat his cancer and preserve his racing career simultaneously—a no compromises, take-no-prisoners approach. Even a famous celebrity like Lance learned that doctors are different and there really isn't only one way to address any given cancer. He got different answers, different prognoses and wildly different recommendations. When choosing your own Cancer, Inc., it's important that you select and direct a team to meet your objectives.

Still, most people don't have the luxury to doctor shop. Lance was single with no kids and he had considerable resources; he was able to fly and set up camp away from home for his care. This option isn't available to most of us. Most people go to their community hospital or medical practice and are assigned a doctor; unless there is a problem, they take what they get. People with good insurance who live near a major metropolitan area may look for a famous medical institution with a "good brand" and commute for their cancer treatment. Others with means use Google to figure out the best place for their cancer type and get themselves to faraway famous hospitals like MD Anderson, the Mayo Clinic, Boston General, Johns Hopkins and Memorial Sloan Kettering Cancer Center—these people are known as medical tourists.

I think there are several considerations before deciding which approach is right for you and there are some creative hybrid options that don't occur to most people. But this isn't the deli counter; you shouldn't just take a number and agree to be served by whoever steps up first. This is probably the most important decision you will make. Most people spend more time researching the performance, features, available brands and best place to buy a DVD player than they do when going to get treatment for a life-threatening disease. Unfortunately, not all doctors and care facilities are the same. The number one variable correlating with survival for my cancer type was whether you were treated in a high-volume dedicated sarcoma unit. Where you go for treatment definitely matters.

*"Famous Brands" versus community hospitals*

There is some controversy in the cancer community about the big "brand" hospitals versus community-based care and there's no right answer. If I were 120 years old with inoperable pancreatic cancer, personally I'd stay at home to enjoy my remaining time. If I were the parent of a child with a rare but beatable sarcoma, I'd go for specialized care wherever it is if I could swing it. It, of course, depends on the situation and on your personal values and needs. The cold reality of cancer is that it is not egalitarian and no health scheme being debated will change that. Most people simply can't pick up their family and set up camp in some faraway city for the extended and ongoing care required for cancer. Some patients are just not stable and cannot travel. Lance left Austin, Texas for care in Indianapolis, but many of us have no option but to accept what's available in our neighborhood.

Even if you are lucky enough to live near a "big brand" hospital you can't just walk in off the street. Some restrict patient transfers by ambulance; you need to be well enough to walk in or have a physician arranged hand-off. Other times they tell you the first available consult is weeks or even months away and they require all kinds of documents and data filed in advance just for the initial consult. If you're lucky enough to pass all these gates, you will be amazed to see how unequal medical care can really be. MSKCC in New York has many high-roller cancer tourists. Russian men with drivers arrive en masse, Japanese, Europeans and a family up from Texas, they're all there. Many big name hospitals even have an international patient system that turnkey manages their special needs. All you need is a credit card prepayment and you're in. This isn't an option for many families and sadly, most need to go to the local hospital or oncology practice and hope that the team that is available is up to the job. Usually, that's ok.

If you have an ear infection or appendicitis, any certified care facility in the world can handle it. These are widespread diseases with standard treatment protocols and low variance in outcome. Some cancers are more like that than others are. Unfortunately, breast cancer, colon cancer, skin cancer, and prostate cancer are so widespread that there are very able, excellent care facilities all over the world that can handle them. That's because they all get enough volume to stay "in practice" and the huge volumes of these diseases have created fairly standard treatment protocols and guidelines. Doctors stay current with these diseases as their continuing education, conferences and trade magazines keep these cancers in the spotlight. I still think there's merit to high volume teaching hospitals but if traveling to a big brand isn't an option for you, my personal view is that's ok for these most common cases. I still recommend meeting the team, verifying the surgeon and being active in choosing the specific doctors.

This is less true for more rare or risky cancers like brain tumors, pancreatic cancer, and sarcomas to name a few. There are many subcategories of rare cancers and they require specialized techniques and treatment protocols. Childhood cancers require different medical protocols but also different support mechanisms and child-friendly environments and may require a dedicated children's hospital. Having had a rare cancer that was misdiagnosed for a long time, I strongly recommend that if you have a choice, go to the facility that handles the most volume and avoid a hospital, practice and doctor that haven't managed a reasonable number of your kind of cancer—especially if your cancer is rare.

There are statistically different outcomes for people with difficult cases when they go to well-known teaching hospitals and it does matter. Top-name hospitals attract top talent from all over the world; the best and brightest gravitate to these places, as does the grant money. It's where clinical trials are happening, where the latest equipment is and where the experience that comes with repetition comes from. My local medical facility had never seen a Ewing Sarcoma before and even a major university teaching hospital in Philadelphia felt they weren't the best nearby team and recommended I go 90 miles up the road to MSKCC for better survival odds. If it's risky and you can shop, you should.

*Cancer is not a "one-off" procedure*

If you have a risky or rare cancer and find you need to travel to a specialized facility, you have problems and special considerations. Cancer requires total care integration and long-term ongoing follow-up; it's not cut and run. Because most patients can't relocate permanently near their specialty medical center, they usually go there for surgery and a treatment plan and then back home for the more standard stuff like chemo. Sometimes they stay for the treatment but return home for ongoing follow-up with a local oncologist while keeping the out-of-town specialist updated. I call this "a la carte cancer management" and it can work and may be the only viable option for some people.

Still, it is extremely difficult to manage cancer treatment this way and it introduces risk and heavy administrative burdens. Many care facilities vertically integrate and have systems and tools that connect the pathologists, x-ray technicians, lab workers, surgeons and oncologists. In spite of assurances otherwise, it can be very difficult to take your surgical notes and CT scans out of San Antonio and get Cancer, Inc in California to deal with it, trust me. Even routine things are very difficult. When you have cancer, there is constant lab work and blood to draw…literally a 30-second nurse meeting. MSKCC was a 90-minute train and subway commute for me just for a pinprick. To save myself stress, I tried to just get my blood drawn close to my home from a local practice but the hospital was very reluctant to use that to clear me for chemotherapy. I had to work the phones and fax to get the blood test result from my local doctors to MSKCC in the right format, to the right people, on time to clear me for procedures.

While it's all possible, the hospital bureaucracy can tend to kill off "outside" procedures and make it hard to let them enter into their world. Do not underestimate the complex, integrated project management that is needed if you try to involve multiple parties on your own. I happened to get my surgery done "outside" at a Philadelphia hospital and they also did some initial scans. Ultimately, MSKCC ended up doing their own pathology again and their own scans to get things the way they liked them, in their format, on their proprietary system, and networked to all their stakeholders (including the billing department). It can be managed but be aware that it's some work!

I also learned that there is an accountability consideration when you mix and match. You want to avoid having no one "own you." If you "doctor shop" and get your surgery from one place and then move to a local facility for ongoing care (chemo, radiation), while farming out lab work to a local doctor,  there can be a lot of finger pointing. Your local oncologist may feel he can't vouch for surgery done at an "outside facility" and may distance himself from your prognosis. It is critical that you understand this before attempting to put the piece parts together yourself.

Obviously, these issues are of secondary concern. If you have a rare brain tumor or a recurrence and you can swing it, I feel you should get the opinion, expertise and surgery from a place that does 100 per week instead of a community-based hospital that does one every 10 years. If you can't swing it, do extra due diligence on the local options and make sure you have the best team that is available, especially for surgery.

Cancer, Inc. is the organization that will try and save your life. Be active in selecting and directing the team.

# 9

## You Win with the Putter

You've seen it a thousand times on television, Lance sprinting to victory across the finish line with his arms off the handlebars extended in the air. But every race fan knows that the real victory was won in the foothills and on the long grueling climb miles before that finish line. You win golf matches with your putter, not with that big impressive tee-shot; and you win the Tour de France with your roadwork. It's the little things that matter, the fundamentals, not the flash.

It's the same with cancer. After going five rounds with the monster, I figured out there are some fundamentals that apply to every cancer fight. I can't guarantee victory but I can help you stack the odds in your favor, eliminate unnecessary risks, reduce stress and save all-important energy.

*Back to school*

You are about to get an advanced degree with a dual major in medical oncology and hospital administration. It's a good idea to approach it like advanced course work and get yourself organized accordingly. My physical cancer notebook was an "old school" thing of scholastic beauty: a classic three-ring binder with tab sections for each critical treatment subject and disk sleeves to keep CD-ROM copies of PET/CT/MRI scans. On the inside panel of the notebook I taped a contact list that included all addresses and reach numbers for my doctors, nurses, chemotherapy and radiation clinics as well as local pharmacies, insurance agents, taxi services, family members and neighbors.

This notebook came with me for every office visit, trip to the lab, and radiation/chemotherapy treatment. It might be hard for you to imagine now but your doctor may take a great new job in California, you could move or five years later your cancer can recur and without the notebook, you'd waste a lot of energy getting the new team up to speed. My notebook also got me out of several jams during treatment and helped relieve anxiety. I had tabs that focused on five phases of my treatment and I recommend you ask for copies of each of the indicated forms and disks (see figure 2).

There are some very important details in these reports and you will want them for the future but also for management of your treatment plan right now. The various *pathology reports* from the diagnosis phase will decide your future and treatment plan and it's often controversial. You may think that cancer is black and white and definitively classifiable, but it's not true. When you read a pathology report, you'll learn that they are triangulating on the "best-fitting" cancer type based on a series of chemical tests applied to your tumor.

(Figure 2)

| Phase of Treatment | Major Materials to Request |
|---|---|
| **Diagnosis** | <ul><li>Disk copies of CT/MRI/PET</li><li>Radiology reports that summarize findings from the CT/MRI/PET scans and X-Rays.</li><li>Biopsy reports (pathology)<ul><li>Cytology report</li><li>Immunophenotype report</li><li>Genetic tumor tests</li></ul></li><li>Blood test reports (CBC panel)</li><li>Oncology report/treatment plan</li></ul> |
| **Surgery** | <ul><li>Surgical report ("Op Note")</li><li>Surgical pathology report</li></ul> |
| **Radiation** | <ul><li>Radiology treatment plan report</li><li>Post procedure evaluation report</li></ul> |
| **Chemotherapy** | <ul><li>Chemo treatment plan report</li><li>Post-procedure evaluation report</li></ul> |
| **Check-ups and recurring scans** | <ul><li>Consultation report (summary of scan results for CT/MRI/PET)</li><li>Disk copies of recurring scans</li><li>Lab reports (blood, ultrasound)</li></ul> |

It turns out that tumors may not be uniform throughout and could be of a mixed type; or your tumor may mostly react like a certain cancer but not fit its profile perfectly (but better than other choices). The pathologists consider the "differential analysis" by holding your tumor up against the profile of their best other guesses and then they choose the best-fitting culprit. Sometimes, there are wildly different treatment protocols for the other candidates so it's an important call.

You want to read the pathology report and see if there is any controversy and discuss with your doctor the implications of any uncertainty. In my case, the tumor was not classic. It was lacking a known genetic marker (which sometimes happens) but it reacted mostly like Ewing's Sarcoma. In my case, deciding how to proceed was easy because the treatments were the same for most of the other alternatives. We did an extra test at my request to rule out the possibility of lymphoma because it would warrant an entirely different set of drugs and treatment cycles. By reading the pathology report and discussing it with my oncologist, I got extra assurances that we were on the right plan. Trust pathology, but verify.

The *surgical report,* also referred to as the "op note", tells you the technique used to remove your tumor and if the surgeon was able to remove it "en masse" or if it needed to be cut into sections first. It also tells you if he was able to get wide margins. The *surgical pathology report* tells you at exactly what point cancer cells were detected while you were open on the table, where they stopped, and if they were touching anything important. This information will be critical when you discuss radiation and chemotherapy later with other members of Cancer, Inc. I used this report to weigh my risks and I didn't like what I read. There were no wide margins and the cancer was near nerves and glands that could provide convenient highways for microscopic spreading. After receiving my oncologist's *treatment plan* (and the chemo and radiation plan), I intervened and asked to consider a more aggressive approach. I wanted to hedge against the narrow margins and likely microscopic spills and I added rounds of chemotherapy and doses of radiation (which I later backed off slightly).

Each of the five sections in my notebook represents a "decision point" that requires patient involvement for key policy decisions. If you don't participate, Cancer Inc. will decide policy for you and their decisions are not purely medical or technical in nature. There is always a trade-off to make between beating the cancer and taking on collateral damage. Sometimes the bet is short term: should a limb be removed as insurance against cancer recurrence, or should it be salvaged to preserve function? Other times a doctor decides to risk the future to guarantee a short-term remission. A "middle-of-the-road" treatment plan might be established, beyond any criticism either way, but possibly losing on all fronts. Unless you're active in these policy decisions, doctors may deduce your wishes circumstantially: "He's young, better be safe, increase the dose." But it's your choice. You can outsource these policy decisions or get involved; either way it's a decision.

*Beware of the change order*

I know it's amazing with all of the safety procedures and control processes but chemotherapy is not goof-proof and mistakes do occur. That's because it is not a fixed and static plan but something constantly re-evaluated and adjusted based on lab reports, blood levels and patient performance. If your white blood cells are trending too low, the doctor may decide to reduce dosages on a given day or cancel one of the treatments. If you aren't responding well, a new drug might be added, a dosage increased, or a treatment sequence changed. This is usually when the process breaks down and mistakes are made. One day, it happened to me and I ended up missing a very important dosage—like with antibiotics, it's important to maintain a consistent level in your bloodstream but because of the administrative error, I accidentally did a seesaw.

After that, I relied heavily on my three-ring bible. Right there in my chemotherapy tab I had the intended treatment plan. I knew the drugs I was supposed to have, the dosage I was supposed to take and the frequency of the treatments. When the doctor wanted that changed, I recorded it because I knew there could mistakes between his office and the reports followed by the chemo floor days later. On more than one occasion, I relied on my handy binder to be sure I got the right treatment. I know of other chemo patients that got it wrong somewhere along the line too, so it's good to stay on top of it and verify every injection against your own records.

The last and important benefit of my notebook was for anxiety management. 90-day scan reports frequently reported nodules, cysts and other suspicious marks. My notebook provided comfort when I compared those reports to ones from a year earlier and found all the same notations. It's apparently a convention to keep reporting the same things over and over even when they're stable and proven inconsequential. I learned what not to worry about by going through consultation reports, which pile up as you get ongoing check-up scans.

*Modern e-tools*

I was very proud of my "old school" notebook but I'm an IT and telecommunications guy and I knew there were better tools. I regret telling you about the sorry state of e-tools at Cancer, Inc. It is not digital, electronic or modern in any consistent way. Most have a website and some are rolling on e-tools for appointment making; but the vast majority of institutions are stuck in 1985. Want a copy of a scan report, no problem, they'll print it out for you or if you prefer, they'll fax it. Does anyone still have a fax? Want to zap over your MRI report from your local hospital, sorry, Cancer, Inc. needs a disk copy and in their proprietary format. Have a quick question or need a short answer, forget about email/text/voicemail, the doctor returns calls from his landline telephone Wednesday afternoons. Every time you go to another department (surgery, radiology, chemotherapy, oncology, reconstructive surgery...) you fill out the same paper form and answer the same questions even if you return weekly. It's like meeting for the first time every week. I've filled out my 40-year medical history with dates of various surgeries and shots 300 times. Eventually to "hack" the system, I stole a form copy, filled it out once and made 50 photocopies. Let's not even get into insurance claims, billing collections and all the other administrative nonsense dominating our system.

To endure this pre-modern culture, I strongly recommend you buy yourself a scanner and sign up for an online service like e-fax so you can send and receive faxes from anywhere you have internet access. Your doctor and insurance company will want faxes back and forth and you will often be working with paper that you need to digitize. Because you will constantly need to commit to new follow-ups and appointments, have a PDA/smartphone or other electronic calendar so you can make adjustments to your schedule on the fly. I think a small laptop or netbook is an excellent thing to ferry around to your millions of appointments.

Last, many patients are using blogs or social networking sites to keep their community efficiently updated with status, pictures and words of encouragement. While much of Cancer Inc. has not modernized their own back office, they have updated their patient environments with wireless LANs, flat screens and connected work stations. With laptop in hand, I was able during chemo to stay in electronic touch with people back home in Cancerville. I think a webcam is a great idea for all cancer patients. There will be times you can't travel or need to be isolated with low blood counts and a webcam can help you stay connected to the world. Some hospitals even provide a website that you can use for updating supporters about your status.

*The listener advocate*

When the critical phases of your cancer treatment come up, I strongly recommend that you bring someone along with a very special profile. For me, that was Audrey, my sister-in-law. Audrey is a smart, no-nonsense, sophisticated professional and she loves me but with a different lens than my wife or parents. This is the perfect profile; someone who cares a lot but isn't in so deep that she can't process information objectively. You definitely should not attend meetings alone when your diagnosis is being read out or your treatment plan is being discussed, and your spouse may be just as emotional and overwhelmed as you.

At my first meeting, the oncologist tried to be very encouraging and said, "We'll beat this, Ewing's has a very high cure rate." Emotionally that was wonderful to hear and my man-pride prevented me from showing any fear or doubt about it. Audrey wasn't so easily persuaded. "But Scott read on the internet that only about half make it five years." Audrey knew I would suffer all the way home trying to reconcile the doctor's statement with what I had read. Better to get it out on the table.

The doctor went on to validate the 50% risk but explained why he thought my situation was better than average. By having someone there who knew my questions and worries, I was able to get a richer learning about my situation and clarity that I alone wasn't able to extract. When you are emotional and dealing with your own possible death, it is very difficult to be competent and systematic. If you have access to one, get yourself an "Audrey" before each key phase of cancer treatment begins (and also during follow-up scans).

*The B-Team*

If Cancer, Inc. isn't in your immediate local community, get a local oncologist who works within a few miles of your home. MSKCC was a bridge, tunnel and train ride away—a 90-minute commute from my home in New Jersey under the best of conditions. Something can go wrong at any hour and it's smart to plan on the contingency that you can't make the trek into Cancer, Inc. I was transparent with B-Team that they were my backstop and they proved to be a wonderful resource. B-Team was very impressed with my three-ring binder and got a duplicate copy. They were fully briefed and always knew my exact status at any given moment. I kept a recurring office appointment with B-Team just to be sure they were up to date but I found it was also an incredible resource for getting a second opinion about how things were going and to see what they thought about a reading on my latest CT scan. I slept better knowing that I had a neighborhood team and often benefitted from their view of Team-A's progress. Another helpful tip is to always have a bag packed. I had a duplicate set of toiletries, emergency clothes and even a back-up cell phone always ready should we need to jump in the car or ambulance.

*Performance management*

Lance is an expert at this and brought his discipline to cancer treatment too. I strongly recommend every cancer patient puts a classic plan in place with these attributes:

**Milestones and metrics**

Bernice was a master at making charts and graphs to track my progress against the goal. It kept me focused, allowed me to set the right pace and allowed me to break down the enormous task in front of me into manageable and achievable sub-steps. It was important that these tools were graphical and visibly posted for all to see as I got support and reinforcement from family, friends and visitors who would see my status.

### Continuous daily improvement

After key milestones, I reviewed with my doctor how my progress was going and checked my status against the original treatment plan. Together we assessed if we were on the right track and if any adjustment to the plan was warranted. We reviewed things that didn't go well and made adjustments to procedures, administration and communications that weren't perfect.

### Celebrate success, reward and recognize achievement

When I finished a cycle or completed a milestone, my family celebrated. There were dinners out, gifts, cakes and parties. Families can greatly support a cancer patient by helping him mark progress and celebrate achievement.

### Publish results to the team

When I got results from tests and passed key milestones, I updated Cancerville by phone, email and later by Facebook.

### Motivate the team

In Chapter 5, I mentioned the professionals in Cancerville who also have needs. The doctors, technicians, and administrative staff also need encouragement, support and recognition for their contribution to your recovery. I bring the best chocolate in the world (Marcolini Belgian Chocolate) to every office visit; my deal with the staff is they keep giving me good news and I keep bringing the chocolates! When I finished my 34 radiation treatments, I thanked the young, urban-hipster technician staff that helped me every day with gift certificates to Tower Records and Starbucks. My chemo nurses, a true troupe of saints, were heading to Haiti for a medical charity and we brought in bags of clothes for their cause. These were small and inexpensive things but people in a community are supposed to notice the contribution of others and take care of each other too. It's also important that the patient thank his family, friends and support network so they link their support to your recovery and feel good about their contribution. Cancer is a community disease but it's also a team success.

*Go the dentist*

It might be the last thing on your mind after a cancer diagnosis but going to the dentist before starting chemotherapy and radiation will save you a lot of pain and possibly your life too. Chemotherapy often creates lesions in your mouth, eroding gum tissue and exposing weak teeth to risk. Radiation anywhere near the head and neck is also a problem. High-energy beams burn lesions in the mouth and on the tongue and gums, weakening surrounding teeth. So, it's a good idea to get a general cleaning and quick repair of any trouble spots before starting any cancer therapy. Once you are on chemo, a bad tooth can be a serious problem. With white blood cells low, it can be very dangerous getting an abscess or any kind of tooth or gum-related infection. Because of the risks, you may also not be cleared for procedures like tooth removal, root canal, or even drilling and routine fillings during chemo or radiation therapy. It's best to tackle the problem upfront.

*Hand sanitizer and room control*

It's a smart idea to organize your living space to protect you and make things easy. We had hand sanitizer bottles strategically located at all entrances, bedrooms, bathrooms and the kitchen. Anyone who entered the house, including visitors and the cable guy, needed to squirt a dollop of the bacteria killing gel on their hands. Bernice would use Clorox® wipes to attack the doorknobs, telephone, remote controls and light switches several times per day. It's important to not use antibacterial soaps, which can cause resistant bacteria to flourish. Products like Purell® are 62% rubbing alcohol and create no resistant strains; same for Clorox products which rely on bleach to do the job.

I had my own cupboard and refrigerator section, bathroom, toiletries and linens. With a small amount of care, I was able to go an entire year without a major fever or infection in spite of having zero white blood cells for ten days every month. This is a remarkable accomplishment and it was the key to me staying on chemotherapy consistently and out of the emergency room. If you make a small effort with this, you can possibly save your life both by avoiding killer infections and by staying on chemo. If there is any hint of a cold, the oncologists will cancel your next treatment round. Infection will kill you before cancer so they are very draconian about it. If you want to stay on cycle, stay on hand sanitizers. Ninety percent of infections come from your hands. Avoid uncooked food and maintain good personal hygiene. To this day, I keep the ritual going, and am rarely sick, even years later.

*See a lawyer, inventory your assets*

It's the last thing you want to do when you get sick but getting your estate in order is the first thing you need to do. Cancer can go badly quickly and when it does, you may not be in a physical or mental state to make important legal decisions. You must make a will and people with significant assets should consider estate planning to be sure the family is protected in the event of your death. I strongly recommend that life insurance policies get reviewed and family members know what assets exist, where they are, what the account numbers and PINs are for various bank accounts, equities, real estate and insurance plans. It is better to get that organized and ready now than wait until it's an emergency. We had a will already but had the good sense to review it upon my illness. We discovered that our assets had changed and our situation too and some changes were in order. You should always review these items when a new important event like a baby, a divorce or a catastrophic illness hits. No one wants to be talking about these legal and administrative items during one's last days and it's better to get it out of the way.

*Keep a multi-media journal*

Cancer treatment is all about repeating cycles. Over time, you become an expert on how your body reacts and there's a rhythm that starts to set in. I found I would get a low-grade fever on day three after chemo and during that time, my body would flush red where it contacted surfaces. The first time it happened, I stressed and went to the e-room because fever is a big risk for cancer patients. Over time, I learned it would pass and wasn't an emergency. By trial and error, I also learned that I could moderate mouth sores by chewing ice during vincristine infusion. Over time, I could tell you exactly when my white blood cells would bottom and the day they would start to rebound. I started to learn which foods would tempt nausea and which ones kept me solid.

I strongly recommend that you keep a journal, especially during the early days to keep track of what happens and at what intervals. This helps manage anxiety and gives you a toolkit to mark your progress and control variables that can help you. I also suggest you take many digital photos of your treatment area but also of your entire body, especially around lymph nodes, eyes, head and neck, and trunk. Be sure they are date stamped and consider taking them again from the same angle at regular intervals. It is very helpful have a digital baseline of your body because over the course of your treatment, you may notice changes that concern you and you'll want to be able to compare to an earlier time. This is especially helpful if you suffer from "scanxiety" (see Chapter 7) and think you notice a new bump or raised area or something else different. For me, the photos often proved my own paranoia and I was able to avoid an office visit or another scan.

*Take a break*

Lance doesn't always train. He enjoys having a drink, traveling, going to restaurants and hanging around with friends, and he's still a world champion! You don't have to dedicate your life to cancer management alone. Part of a good training program is stepping away from the grind once in awhile. I found it very helpful to buy some new nice clothes, go to a spa, have a luxurious trip, and go fishing with my kids. I was able to recharge my batteries and stay focused. I found regular, light exercise to be wonderful, especially playing tennis and riding the bike. It clears the mind and gives you a sense that you are still alive physically and investing in your body. It's a great idea to visit with friends and take small trips if you can.

# 10

# The Power and Price of Google!

When Lance got his cancer in 1996, there were just 36 million internet users and it was still two years before the technical launch of Google.[8] It's amazing how much everything has changed. Lance writes about becoming a student of cancer and it was definitely an old school approach! "I went to the biggest bookstore in Austin and bought everything there on the subject," he writes, and then describes how he learned everything he could so he could actively participate in his treatment decisions. He read back issues of *Yoga Journal* and scoured pages of *Discover* magazine; it almost seems quaintly antique by today's standards. Lance then toured the country and interviewed experts to understand his disease, prognosis and treatment options.

It's a very different game today. Now there are more than 1.5 billion internet users and Google has become a standard verb. Everything about your disease is on the web and your oncologist probably hates that. You can get raw data from clinical trials just completed in France and abstract reports telling you what they mean. You can learn what causes your cancer and, if you have the patience, you can learn about the molecular signature of your cancer, its fusion subscript characteristics and the immuno-histological chemical reactions that can help identify and classify it. There's a treasure trove of information about the latest thinking in treatment strategies and documented medical debates about the ideal frequency, sequencing and thresholds of radiation and chemotherapy needed to fight your exact cancer type.

*Trying to calculate the "odds"*

Most modern cancer patients spend time on Google trying to handicap our chances. It's right there in black and white: prognosis statistics. Google will tell you the percent of people with your disease that make it five years and you can read about the variables that correlate with survival and how big of an influence they have. Was your tumor over two centimeters, was there more than 50% necrosis, was it located on the head or neck…add a point here, subtract one there…you can start to triangulate on your odds. The statistics are to four decimal places so it seems pretty sure.

All of this information is misleadingly accessible but often its complexity, meaning and accuracy are masked. As any doctor can attest, oncology in the post-Google era means they are dealing with patients newly armed with detailed information but not necessarily experience, knowledge or training to interpret it. The statistics can be tricky. Many of the statistics are about disease-free survival rates, which are different from survival rates (many people battle cancer chronically for decades). Many cancer types affect very old people or people with other diseases who already have low five-year survival rates. And making it five years can mean you'll make thirty, there's a lot not said in these statistics.

Also, a lot of the data is old. There have been huge gains in drugs, radiation therapy, nausea control, and early recurrence detection—and it's a big deal. The impact of these developments is often not found in the 5-10 year survival averages published on the web. If a drug dosage or sequence change is found today to improve patient response, it will take five years to get a study funded that will have to run ten years before the improvement rate is documented. That's 15 years of lagging data. MSKCC has, for years, been doing its own protocol for treating my cancer type because they see many cases and have evidence that a higher dosage but shorter duration program works best. I might already be on a different survival trajectory than the data indicates on Google.

Bottom line: "survival rate" information on the web is not intended to tell you your chances. It's used for technical people to compare long term trends over very long periods of time. It has little to do with your prognosis and most of the studies are at least 15 years old. Don't let prognosis statistics upset you, they never look positive!

*How to use Google with your doctor*

In the post-Google era, the best oncologists recognize that they have motivated, self-educated, patient-partners who will have opinions and a desire to participate in their treatment decisions. Sometimes these patient-partners have new information and good ideas—because of Google! The best patients recognize that having a web browser is no substitute for their doctor's decades of training and they listen and trust the final advice from their doctor. The best arrangement should be a partnership of mutual respect that works like that.

My research showed data out of Europe that radiation over a certain amount did not improve outcomes in Ewing's Sarcoma but did significantly raise the risk of radiation induced new cancers. My treatment plan was designed to go past that important threshold and I brought the study in to discuss it. My doctor team was wonderful. They weren't defensive or dismissive and treated my information with interest. They felt I should risk a new cancer down the road in order to beat this one aggressively—the excess radiation raised the risk but it was still single-digit probability. The current cancer was a clear and present danger and they felt better whacking it hard. We compromised and backed the plan below the risk threshold but still higher than what the standard protocol called for. It was an open, collaborative, and fact-based team decision. You want to go for this kind of dynamic with your cancer team.

Because oncologists know that Google is not always their friend, unless you ask, many will keep surgical notes, pathology reports, blood tests and follow-up scan reports to themselves. They may prefer to tell you how you're doing instead of giving you raw data for you to make your own assessment. Google doesn't just mislead you about prognosis; it can also cloud the meaning of these routine reports. There's also something very difficult for scientists to admit: the best doctors know when to worry and when not to worry based on their cumulative experiences and intuitive impression of your specific case, which means their "art" can sometimes over-rule the "science" written in various technical reports. Sometimes a good oncologist knows something but can't tell you why his life experiences guide him to that conclusion; raw report data can obscure this ability.

Google told me that the high "standard uptake value" (SUV) in my thyroid PET scan was almost statistically certain to be a cancer recurrence. The scan report that is conventionally written in cold, binary language certainly gave no comfort: "High SUV is above critical threshold at thyroid; recommend clinical evaluation to rule out cancer recurrence." I read this after my oncologist gave me an "all clear" in person with smiles and congratulations and sent me on my way with euphoria. How could he tell me I was fine with such an elevated SUV?!

The region in question was adjacent to my original tumor and seemed an obvious location for a recurrence risk. What was going on here?

When I called my doctor to understand this, he told me not to worry about it, that he was right and just trust him because he knew it was simple inflammation, "thyroditis". He told me the guys who write up the reports need to be binary and there's a convention about what to say but that his job was to interpret that and he was comfortable all was fine.

Always a fan of the "trust but verify" principle, I wanted to know the rationale behind his conclusion. And then I was humbled. I'm a smart guy, I read a hundred reports online and deluded myself into thinking I was fairly competent. My doctor knew I was suffering acid reflux, he had seen the radiation report and knew the thyroid was in the exit beam zone. He had (unknown to me) been tracking intervals of up and down swings on the thyroid before and looking into blood tests and other data. "It doesn't fit a cancer profile the way it came on anyway and with all the radiation you did; nothing will come back in that location, especially not now after this short time. If we have a problem, it will be in your lungs." He knew this PET scan reading was "noise" and didn't think twice about it. It's why they don't like to release the raw reports for us layman to suffer over.

I asked him about the "clinical evaluation" recommended in the scan report so he acquiesced and ordered an ultrasound. Conclusion: "thyroiditis". Since that incident, I've had a pain behind my surgical-side eye, a lump appeared on the palm of my hand, and I had deep bone pain in a leg. According to Google, these things were all very worrying given my specific disease. I was constantly amazed at how my oncologist was bored by these developments and sure it wasn't a concern. He had more reasons than he could explain as to why he wasn't worried. He knew from 20 years of experience and by triangulation of variables in his mind. These symptoms, in isolation, were worrying, but he had reasons for why they didn't fit a recurrence scenario for my specific case given their timing, location, presentation, and given scan results from just 90-days before. My oncologist always proved right and I was always quite surprised how he could know.

*Use Google for questions, not answers*

I strongly recommend patients rely on the web only to guide questions and to improve understanding of what the doctors say. I strongly advise against using it to make conclusions especially about one's prognosis or the right treatment plan. If my tumor was a half-centimeter to the right, it would have invaded a critical nerve (a super highway for metastasis) and entered my parotid gland offering easy access to lymph nodes and circulatory systems. Lucky for me, the tumor was a half-centimeter to the left in a relatively benign bed of fat and soft tissue. That means my prognosis and treatment plan were wildly affected by a half centimeter and Google just can't capture that. Every cancer is individualized and you have your very own survival probability; the way you respond to treatments and the meaning of test results are also greatly individualized.

When you pass through the five key decision phases of cancer treatment (see Chapter 9), use Google to bone up on the right issues and considerations to discuss with your doctor team before you lock down on treatment policy and strategy. It took awhile but eventually I stopped trying to have the web divine my future and I even stopped verifying my doctor's conclusions after every check up! Eventually I realized that all the checking wasn't giving me more peace or comfort. It took me three years to notice that the doctor knew better, every time. I regret the energy wasted doubting and checking everything he said. I'm a telephone company guy, not a medical oncologist, and broadband internet doesn't change that. Use the web to get informed but leave it at that. Find an oncologist who you are comfortable with and let him help you with what it all means. They have medical school for a reason.

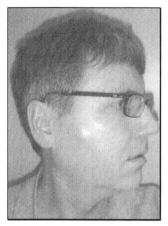

**Photo 1:** Lump, day before surgery

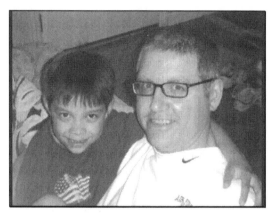

**Photo 2:** Dad and Gavin "before"

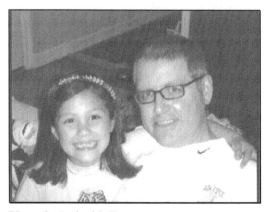

**Photo 3:** And with Zoe

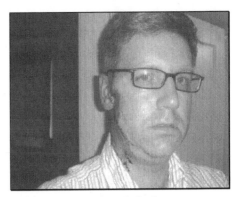

**Photo 4:** Three days "after"

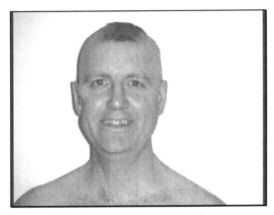

**Photo 5:** Obligatory Chemo Mohawk

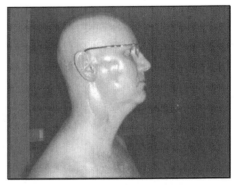

**Photo 6:** Full toxic state after chemo

**Photo 7:** First day back to work

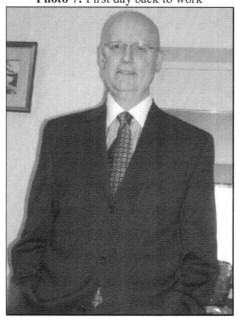

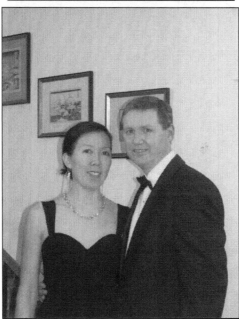

**Photo 8:** Bernice and me, 1-year remission

# 11

# New Age Miracles and the Lost Establishment

When Lance learned about the toxic damage that chemo would do to his body, his instinct was to fight it; he was a highly tuned world-class athlete and his body was something worth preserving.

After consulting a local nutritionist, Lance decided on his diet: "a lot of free-range chicken, broccoli, no cheeses or other fats and a lot of vitamin C to help combat the toxins of chemo."

Many patients try to do the same. Today, there is a treasure trove of solutions on the internet to block the damage of radiation and chemotherapy and people are self-medicating with megadoses of everything from shark cartilage to maitake mushrooms. Particularly popular are megadoses of vitamins, anti-oxidants, amino acids, hormones, and concentrated green tea extracts. Usually, the websites selling these solutions point to millennia of use in China or to a non-peer-reviewed study done by a professor in Japan or Argentina that "proves" its efficacy. The problem is the entire point of radiation and chemotherapy is to poison your cells and it may be counterproductive to try to block that.. The American Cancer Society gives a very sober caution about all of this:

"Some people with cancer take large amounts of vitamins, minerals, and other dietary supplements in an effort to enhance their immune systems or even destroy cancer cells. Some of these substances can be harmful. In fact, large doses of some vitamins and minerals may reduce the effectiveness of chemotherapy and radiation therapy".[9]

In fact, a very long and formal study out of USC was just in the news proving that green tea blocks the effectiveness of many important chemotherapy agents especially in a class of important new cancer drugs called proteasome inhibitors. "The most immediate conclusion from our study is the strong advice that patients undergoing cancer therapy with (this class of drugs) must avoid green tea, and in particular all of its concentrated products that are freely available from health food stores,"[10] advised the lead researcher.

Many patients today are taking enormous vitamin C supplements before, during and after chemotherapy treatments. But a study undertaken by Dr. Mark Heaney and colleagues at the Memorial Sloan-Kettering Cancer Center in New York published findings in 2008 showing that vitamin C supplements may reduce the efficacy of some of the most common and important cancer drugs including Gleevec®, doxorubicin, cisplatin, methotrexate, and vinscristine.    Incidentally, Lance did a lot of one of those drugs (cisplatin) and I did two of the others. "I don't recommend taking supplemental vitamin C during that period of time that my patients are receiving chemotherapy," Dr. Heaney advised.

There are numerous other studies finding that these massive supplements, herbs and compounds actually reduce or eliminate the effectiveness of chemotherapy and radiation therapy. Megadoses of the popular supplement, St. John's Wort, have been shown to reduce the effectiveness of the important colon cancer drug Camptosar by a whopping 40%, for example.[11]

I'm not trying to discredit alternative medicine, herbs and non-western therapies. On the contrary, it turns out that most industrial chemotherapy drugs come from exotic plants and herbs that have been used for centuries in faraway places for disease management. Eli Lilly's blockbuster chemotherapy drug Oncovin® is actually refined from the Madagascar periwinkle plant where it was used for centuries as a folk remedy. The powerhouse chemotherapy agent doxorubicin attacks lymphoma, sarcomas, leukemia and many other cancers; its heritage comes from some pioneering Italian scientists that noticed the clinical power of microbes in the soil around a 13th century castle in Castel del Monte. Lance's life-saving drug, cisplatin, was bumped into while performing electrolysis of platinum-based electrodes. We should respect these "alternative" secrets and avoid arrogant dismissal of folk remedies.

There are also some pretty solid studies showing that antioxidants in particular may be very beneficial to preventing cancer in the first place. And other studies show that if you mix exactly the right alternative medicine with exactly the right chemotherapy agent at exactly the right interval and dosages, sometimes good things do happen. Green tea extracts for example seem to increase absorption of doxorubicin by cancer cells without increasing concentration in healthy cells; provided it's administered correctly.[12]

The cancer community seems divided ideologically and there's a large group that derides any solution that doesn't come from a drug company with brand name and trademarked logo. My view is to respect vitamins, herbs and other alternatives as legitimate medicines but that's where I part company with the alternative medicine enthusiasts. You would never just pull a chemotherapy drug randomly off the shelf and dose yourself up with it; so you shouldn't, without advice, load up on a megadose of alternative medicines either. Just because something is "natural" doesn't mean it's safe and it absolutely can interact badly with other medicines.

I'm not against herbs and supplements; I'm just against self-medicating and mixing powerfully interacting agents without consideration. If you plan to dose yourself up on something, please check with your doctor first. Sometimes it's ok but many times it's not, and the consequences can be severe.

*Miracle diets and shaman nutritionists*

Isn't it time we finally admit that nutrition isn't a science but something closer to a cult? There are militant adherents to the religion of every dietary obsession you can think of and many of the most militant have PhDs, titles and websites…and they all disagree with each other. They even disagree with themselves over time. The official nutrition advice given to schoolchildren in the shape of a food pyramid reads like a verdict from God. The stability and permanence of the pyramid image seems to reinforce the solidity of the science and the specificity of recommending three servings of this but only two of that make it seem very refined and exact.

Unfortunately, the food pyramid changes like the weather. When I was a kid, the food pyramid seemed to like milk, eggs and meat a lot more than when I became a young adult. All of that then became criminalized for its fat and protein focus so grains, pasta and carbohydrates seemed to be the new secret. Butter and lard was tossed overboard for margarine and olive oil and somewhere down the line, sugar was replaced with high fructose corn syrup and we got flooded with polyunsaturated fats. By my thirties, everyone was worried about the fast starch burn from carbohydrates and after flirting with various grapefruit diets, the Zone, and Atkins, everyone jumped on the protein wagon again. That's until the Lipitor people criminalized cholesterol and declared almost every one of us sick (and a candidate for statins). This isn't a science, it's a fad. Here's a secret, there is no correct universal nutrition formula. And what exactly is a "serving" anyway and how do I know when I ate one? Everyone's metabolism and absorption rates vary and there's absolutely no evidence that if you and I eat exactly the same thing that we get similar outcomes at all on anything you want to measure—serum cholesterol levels, lipids, blood pressure, weight, or body mass index. So what to do? It seems logical to eat a balanced diet which means not including or excluding anything in the extreme and that goes for you meat-only Atkins extremists and your vegan-only friend from college. You're probably both malnourished! Prepare and eat foods slowly instead of buying them processed and don't beat yourself up if you have that ice cream once in awhile. But that's just my non-expert opinion.

If you want to find out what the real experts say you should eat during cancer treatment, forget it. Just go ahead and try and Google the subject. There are thousands of authoritative declarations from experts who say precisely the opposite of each other all over the web. Some want you to eat fat and protein; others want you to never touch that. Some want you to take high calorie drink supplements while others explicitly exclude that. Some recommend replacing lost fluids and electrolytes with sports drinks; others say that will kill you. It's truly mind numbing. I find nutrition to be like cable news—everyone watches the network that affirms his or her existing world view. Nearly every cancer patient I met has chosen the nutrition ideology that fits best with his preconceived notions and defends it as the only true religion in a world of infidels. It's fatiguing watching people say and "prove" opposite and contradicting things.

Because oncologists are practical doctors that have grown up data driven, they tend to avoid the nutrition hype. Or maybe it's because they've learned this is a religious subject for many patients and no matter what they recommend, they can't win. Whatever the reason, I find most oncologists stay in a very safe harbor on this subject. Nearly every oncologist will tell you to eat whatever you want with the main goal being to maintain weight. Cancer treatment grinds you down and if you fall below critical mass, you can lose reserves needed to endure the treatment. This is a problem for the oncologist so he'll encourage you to do whatever it takes to prevent wasting.

Oncologists also tell you to listen to your body. Chemo and radiation kill certain blood cells and bone factories that produce them and many patients find they are craving meat and other rich protein sources to replenish these factories. Like a pregnant woman craving what she needs, it's a good idea to feed the body what it's telling you it wants. Many agree that protein is important while wasting away on chemo. The only other advice is to avoid uncooked food (sushi, fresh fruit, and vegetables) during those treatment times when white blood cells are low. Because there is a fundamentalist cult that believes those are the world's healthiest foods, this annoys many people; but without white blood cells, bacteria on these uncooked foods can kill you.

When you get cancer, your best bet is to leave militant food ideology at the hospital door. Eating will be unappetizing and nauseating anyway so you no longer have the luxury to be picky or ideological. Think of it as "Thai prison time" and yes, eventually, you will eat the cockroach in your cell—even if you're a vegetarian! When it's an emergency, you can't be picky; and cancer is an emergency.

In Chapter 4, I write about doubling my calories just to maintain body weight. In my case, what my body wanted and needed was clear: foods rich in protein and calories. While I continued to eat a balanced diet, I added back things that I was previously restricting because of high cholesterol. Specifically eggs, cheese, and meats of all kinds took on a bigger part of my dietary mix. My body cried for these things and I felt stronger when I put them in my system, so I listened to my body. Because the rest of my family didn't share my caveman dietary focus and because I often became hungry between meals, I found myself planning, shopping for and preparing many of my own feasts!

For reasons I can't explain, after chemotherapy and the "wrong diet" my cholesterol level is now low and stable. It's as if the treatment somehow shocked me into a new state where my body is consuming my serum cholesterol instead of letting it cake up on my artery walls. I've often wondered if the chemo created a nutritional deficit for cholesterol that is now being fed.

*Unregulated Clinics and Miracle Cures*

Lance recalls perusing a pamphlet about the *Clinic of the Americas in the Dominican Republic* which described "an absolutely certain cure for cancer." There's a quite a bit of medical tourism going on now. For $20,000 cash, you can get a supposed tumor suppression gene injected into your arteries at an unregulated clinic in Beijing. "Medical entrepreneur" Neil Riordan is setting up the Institute for Cellular Medicine in Costa Rica to test stem cell therapies away from the heavy hand of the FDA. An impressive number of alternative cancer treatment clinics in Mexico keep getting shut down for lacking papers or for practicing without licenses and experimenting with unproven or disproven treatments. An equally impressive number re-open under new names. The Oasis of Hope is located in Playas de Tijuana, Mexico, and markets itself to stage four cancer patients in America. It offers "body, mind and spirit medicine" thirty minutes from the San Diego airport (but out of regulatory reach). Oasis deploys alternative strategies like ozone therapy, vitamin C and K megadose therapy, and they even give you live bacteria pills to colonize your colon with microbes—they see this as an immune system spark plug of sorts.

I get 2.2 million hits when I Google "miracle cancer cure" and 36 million more for "cancer cure". The websites I read tend to lean towards natural Chinese herbs and food products that "definitively cure all kinds of cancer no matter what stage". Usually the claims are endorsed by a serious-sounding doctor or professor with seemingly legitimate credentials. There's another variety that takes a conspiracy bent usually claiming the industrial medical complex or the U.S. government is holding back the cure. Here are three typical claims:

> "Discover the hidden secret—10 step formula to cure any form of cancer—guaranteed!!!

> "One of the latest 'miracle' cancer cures hails from China, and it is Kanglaite, a preparation made from a traditional staple food. It highlights the nature of Chinese remedies and the Chinese approach to health. Dr. Mae-Wan Ho reports."

> "Here's the miracle cancer cure the FDA does not want you to have! A new medical magic bullet, Antineoplaston therapy, is curing cancers at an astonishing rate – amazingly, the FDA wants to suppress it!"

Like with any business, there are crooks out there and it's a mistake for me to lump all of these companies and offshore institutions into one lot. America's medical approval process is conservative and designed with a bias to defend and protect more than it is to experiment and go fast. There may very well be breakthrough things happening in places more willing to just inject first and ask questions later. For many cancer patients, they don't have the time for a 10-year drug approval process. I've met well-educated and wealthy parents who very rationally say, "What do we have to lose?" when they go for a "Hail Mary" pass offshore in Costa Rica, Thailand, China and Mexico. Isn't it worth $20k to find out? Unfortunately, it's that very condition that causes con artists and hope-peddlers to see cancer families as an easy mark and they prey upon desperate people in hopeless situations.

As a rule of thumb, if someone claims to have "cured cancer" enormous skepticism is due. If someone tells you he believes "cancer" will be cured in a few years, enormous skepticism is due. That's because there is no such thing as cancer. It isn't a monolithic thing; it's like saying they will cure "sickness" in a few years. What does that mean? There are more than 200 different broad types of cancer and hundreds of thousands of subtypes within those categories each with different genetic compositions, their own chromosomal translocations, fusion proteins and cell characteristics. The various cancers out there deploy wildly different cell proliferation strategies and react differently to various compounds and treatment protocols. Yes, we can beat breast cancer tomorrow but it most likely will have no impact on leukemia and colon cancer. It just isn't the same disease.

Lance and I seem to be of the same mind on this. He was treated in Indiana and resisted the "certain cure" waiting for him in the Dominican Republic.

*The lost establishment*

While there are obvious pitfalls chasing the miracle offshore cure and unregulated self-prescribed compounds, not everything is going well in Cancer, Inc. either. When you join the cancer community, your first surprise is how uninterested people seem to be in learning from your case. I considered myself to be a wonderful laboratory rat. Because I was nationally rare getting this disease, I saw myself as a "control group". Very few patients in America get a Ewing's Sarcoma tumor as an adult, without any of the known gene translocations, on the face, and not involving bone. It seemed to me that by being such a rare case, there was a chance to isolate on what was different about me. I hoped my case could shed some light on what caused this unique outcome and that it could be helpful to a more broad population.

And there was something different about me that I thought was fundamental and useful for creating a cure. In spite of twenty years of good health and no significant other medical problem, since birth, I've suffered from chronic autoimmune diseases, a condition that runs in my family. It started out with a state of constant infection. I had six ear infections per year growing up, annual bronchitis and multiple bouts of pneumonia. In my adolescence I developed psoriasis, a disease caused by an over-stimulated immune system. Later I got another rare autoimmune sickness called ITP; essentially, you start bleeding because an overactive and confused immune system starts attacking blood platelets thinking they are foreign substances. All of this stopped by my early teenage years except for the psoriasis, which remained chronic but very moderate; I leave it untreated with little symptoms. Others in my family suffer from Lupus, arthritis, allergies and asthma and both sides of the family have high incidence of these autoimmune disorders.

I have the sense that my immune system went into overdrive triggered by early childhood infections and ever since it's been in a frenzied state attacking various things indiscriminately while missing other important things during the chaos. I think I got cancer because my immune system was distracted, compromised, wrongly focused and not productive. Everyone has cancer cells in their body multiple times during their lives. You probably have some floating around your body right now. Cancer cells are flawed and weak, and because they are different, they have a difficult time binding to other cells and surviving. They are inefficient and require substantial energy to replicate, which means they need to hold on tight and eat huge amounts just to survive. This is why cancer fails routinely and why most people remain disease free. Even if the cells bind and start to replicate, a healthy immune system can hunt down these early-stage tumors and kill them off before trouble begins. My theory is that my own immune system was too busy fighting too many fronts of a war. With sirens blaring and red-alert lights flashing, the cancer enemy snuck in behind distracted defenses.

No one at Cancer, Inc. cared about this at all. It didn't matter. It didn't change what they needed to do. This was a pattern, if it didn't affect the plan, it didn't matter. In fact, in spite of the gains in genetic analysis of tumors, it didn't really matter if my tumor was Ewing's, PNET or Rhabdomyosarcoma—our ability to sub-classify tumors with different genetic structures is beyond our ability to do anything different with that detailed information. We all get the same chemo anyway (chemo that's been around for 40 years). I got the distinct impression that Cancer, Inc. was divided into two worlds: the taskmasters that pack you with 40-year old therapies and the researchers behind microscopes and controlled clinical trials. I got the sense they were somehow institutionally detached from each other.

The linkage between cancer and immune system disorders is not a new idea. There are therapies now and new ideas under development (including from those unregulated new age hospitals in Mexico). The cancer research community is looking into this area at their own pace, with their own experiments and with their own controlled patient studies. Still, I couldn't help but feel that the answer to cancer was walking into to doctors offices every day; plain to see, isolatable common causes just sitting there, detailed on the case history forms we all fill out before every appointment, but that no one seems to read. Are we missing the forest for the trees?

*Where are you Albert Einstein?*

People have a similar reflection in another field of science. The leading physicist of all time was by all accounts bad at math and a poor student; but he unlocked more secrets of the universe than anyone before him or since. Einstein did that by simple thought experiments and representational thinking. He was able to solve big, complex mysteries with simple tangible models. The Big Bang theory, the nature of time and space, and the origins of our universe all come out of Einstein's simple representational thinking.

When I was ill and reading lots of books on philosophy, origins of the universe and physics, I learned that there is a group of scientists who feel we've been on the wrong track ever since Einstein. In his book, *The Trouble with Physics,* Lee Smolin writes about the more than 1,000 researchers worldwide going deeper down a blind alley called "String Theory" and he's worried that theoretical physics is stuck. By his analysis, since Einstein, we've had two generations of physicists getting further away from a unified theory and further away from comprehending our universe. They are lost in minutiae trying to unravel the DNA of the cosmos, trapped at the micro level studying exotic nano-particles, string theory and quantum mechanics. Einstein asked big questions and found big universal truths. Today's physicists are busy looking at the atomic and sub-atomic particle levels. They're looking for the universe's source code and are seeking knowledge from exotic equations. But the more they go deep, the less they learn and the more questions come up. It's a wonderful dark hole to jump in if you're an academic; it's a treasure trove of endless research projects with one door opening yet another in a series of infinite questions. But some feel there is no real new learning, just more data and more questions.

To this layman, cancer research seems at risk of following the same path. There are incredible developments happening especially as we have opened the door to genetic engineering, biology's equivalent to quantum mechanics. Pathology used to decide what kind of tumor you had by staining it with chemicals and seeing how proteins and antibodies reacted to it—an imperfect and qualitative science. Today, that immune-histological classification system is backed up by genetic analysis—a binary and exacting approach. I think about it as cancer going from analog to digital. The idea is that by going "digital", we will comprehend the source code of various cancers and ultimately, we'll make a software fix and re-code whatever is wrong in the human operating system.

*Regressions*

I know a lot about operating systems, digital networks and complex code; it's what I do for a living. "Cancer" shows up all the time in complex IT systems but we call them bugs. Whenever you try to open up source code to fix a bug, you usually get something called a regression. If you work in a company big or small, you know about this. It's when the IT guys try to improve the billing system but instead, the CEO's telephone stops working or the fire alarm goes off every hour! In complex systems, the interdependencies and unknown links only come apparent after the change is implemented. It's the same in complex biological systems. Psoriasis is an annoying and sometimes unattractive affliction but it's chronic and not life threatening. The new drug, Alefacept, is effective at controlling this annoying affliction by suppressing the immune system but it also causes sore throat, dizziness, cough, nausea, itching, muscle aches, chills, injection site pain and injection site redness and swelling. The most serious side effects are a reduction in the number of immune cells, infections, cancer and allergic reactions. That's quite a regression just to reduce an unsightly rash! It's hard to turn something off without turning something else on in complex systems. A single human body is infinitely more complex than the entire wired world. Are we sure we're going to be switching off cancer cells without regression?

When something goes wrong in a telecom or IT network, the best minds from Silicon Valley and Bangalore are very reluctant to open up the middleware and core code of the affected system; they know there is an infinite amount of regressions waiting no matter what variable they manipulate. Experience tells them they can fix the problem but not without creating twenty new problems. They rarely even try. I wish cancer doctors would get together with network operators and systems engineers. Maybe something good would come out of it. I have a few observations about the different philosophies between these communities:

- Oncologists try to kill cancer and win an unconditional surrender. Systems engineers try to quarantine bad code from doing more harm.

- Oncologists try to beat cancer while keeping the patient alive. Systems engineers most effective strategy is to shut down systems (let them die) and reboot later.

- Systems engineers proactively ping networks and know "real time" when software or hardware bombs. Oncologists are reactive or rely on interval screening.

- Systems engineers have a digital copy of the working system and can do a "systems restore" to roll back to an earlier time; oncologists have no digital record of any patient.

- Systems engineers can locate every line of bad code with exhaustive search algorithms; oncologists do full-body scans looking for anomalies and treat the entire body indiscriminately.

My personal opinion is we're a long time away from re-writing human software to correct for cancer bugs without unleashing scary regressions. But I can imagine mass-deployed nano-detection technology that sends an alarm when the first cell goes bad. I can visualize targeted chemotherapy that attacks only cancer cells based on their genetic code. I can imagine therapies that surround early cancer cells behind a firewall allowing them to remain but forever quarantined. And I suspect there is something interesting about killing the human body and re-animating it later as a biological reboot strategy; some kind of controlled cardiac arrest and hypothermia deep-freeze followed by resuscitation. I'm quite optimistic.

I just hope we don't get too lost down there at the molecular level. It's an important moment. Genetic engineering is exciting and it offers a brave new world of novel questions for sharp minds to dive into. But like with physicists, thousands of cancer researchers could go down a blind alley of minutiae and forget to pick their head up for two generations if we're not careful. I suspect we will cure many cancers with a simple and elegant solution that Einstein would be proud of rather than by complexity. Like the concept of warping space/time, the answer to cancer is probably staring at us in the face, just waiting for an "Einsteinian" thinker to be creative enough to see what's right in front of us. And what's in front of us might just be that patient sitting on the table, in a Brooks Brother's Suit, with a case history that tells us something fundamental.

# 12

## Down the Road

Lance finished his treatment nearly 14 years ago. It's inspiring to see him out there today obviously fit and competing against much younger men with great success. He did some serious damage to his body to beat cancer but he seems no worse for the wear. Lance went on to father healthy children and he continues to push his body to incredible limits while competing on the world stage.

Unfortunately, other cancer patients aren't so lucky. We all compromise our future in order to live today. Cancer treatment is toxic and ironically, the treatment itself can cause cancer and many other nasty diseases and conditions. In addition to the immediate problems that come with surgery, chemotherapy and radiation, there are problems that linger called "long-term side effects" and problems that can show up much later called "late side effects".

There's lots of chatter on the web and online discussion groups about late effects. Many people feel they weren't sufficiently warned of problems that might develop or they lack information on what to do and what to look out for to stay ahead of risk. It's important to keep in mind that this subject is a "good problem". If you're worrying about late or lingering side effects, it means you've probably passed the initial challenge and are out of immediate danger from cancer. Many long-term side effects wane over time and the late risks are only potential ones often with incidences in the single-digit percentage range. That's why cancer doctors are willing to take treatment-related risks; beating cancer now far outweighs any concerns about long term (potential) side effects. Here's an abbreviated list of things that can happen compiled mainly from the Mayo Clinic website:

| Treatment | Long-term Side Effects | Late-developing Side Effects |
|---|---|---|
| Surgery | Scars<br>Long-term pain<br>Loss of function | Lymphedema |
| Chemotherapy | Heart failure<br>Kidney failure<br>Liver failure<br>Neuropathy<br>Infertility<br>Menopause<br>Fatigue<br>Chemobrain | Cataracts<br>New primary cancer<br>Lung disease<br>Osteoporosis<br>Hearing loss |
| Radiation | Skin sensitivity<br>Fatigue | Cataracts<br>Tooth decay<br>Thyroid problems<br>Heart problems<br>Lung problems<br>Lymphedema<br>New primary cancer |

Some of these risks are related to specific procedures which have direct impact on targeted areas. Other risks come more often with certain types of drugs. Radiation to the head has a bigger risk on thyroid function than treatment to other areas, for example. Lymphedema happens when surgery or radiation destroys a vital link in the inter-connected lymph system causing fluids to back up and tissues to swell. "Loss of function", described as a surgical risk, is site-specific and the problems can range from infertility (when surgery impacts sexual organs) to mobility problems when limbs are lost. Heart problems come from radiation to the chest and from doxorubicin and cyclophosphamide while lungs are especially challenged by several other popular chemotherapy agents like bleomycin. The risks described as late-developing generally can show up five years or more after the procedure.

So what's a cancer patient to do? Because survival rates are increasing and people with cancer are living longer, it's critical to stay on top of long-term and late-occurring risks. There are special risks for children who survive cancer because late problems can be triggered by the physiological changes that occur with puberty and aging.

You should not assume that your oncologist will automatically set up appropriate screenings for long-term risks. Many patients find doctors dismissive of the entire subject preferring to focus on the more immediate problem at hand. That creates a burden for the patient to monitor the risk areas themselves. Unfortunately, many patients have spent so much time with doctors and hospitals that they choose to turn a blind eye to early warnings from late effects. It's important to stay diligent. Since the risks vary considerably by procedure and drug type, you have to do some homework to monitor your own ongoing risks.

This is where the notebook I described in Chapter 9 becomes critical. You have to know and keep detailed records of the procedures you received, the zones that were treated, the cumulative dosages of each drug type taken and the amount and type of radiation received. With that knowledge firmly in hand, you must read the literature provided by your doctor or find it yourself on the web to know exactly what risks come with your medicine types and procedures.

In general, all recovering cancer patients should focus on healthy living and lowering ongoing risks by not smoking, limiting alcohol and by eating foods rich in calcium and staying fit with moderate exercise. This will help hedge risks for arthritis, joint and connective tissue problems as well as heart, lung and liver disease.

Patients who took drugs or had procedures that put heart function at risk should have regular electrocardiograms (EKG) and echocardiography tests and stay alert for chest pains or tightness. Patients with lung function risk can benefit from imaging scans and lung capacity tests. Blood tests can provide early warning of hormonal imbalances that can be a sign of thyroid dysfunction or damage to the endocrine system which can result from site specific surgery, radiation or certain chemotherapy drugs.

In general, recovering cancer patients should have routine and recurring screenings that assess risk factors specific to the treatment. If this isn't done automatically as part of ongoing care, the patient should take the initiative to ask for and schedule these regular screenings. It is possible that long-term care will be done with new and different doctors who are not part of the cancer management team. Whether it's a cardiologist or a primary care physician doing the long-term care, be sure to hand over your three-ring binder with all your treatments, drug types, dosages and amounts carefully annotated.

I know it's odd to think this way after getting cancer in the first place but I have an odd Darwinian sense about the future. If cancer and cancer treatment didn't kill me, maybe the late effects won't get me either.

# 13

## Obligation of "The Rest"

After his last treatment in 1996, Lance reflected on "the obligation of the cured." He had a new sense of purpose having apparently beaten cancer and he wanted to serve the cancer community. Lance had some business associates research what it takes to start a charitable foundation. He no longer felt his role in life was to be a cyclist but instead saw his role as a cancer survivor. He created the Lance Armstrong Foundation (LAF) with the mission to "inspire and empower cancer sufferers and their families." LAF does everything from raising awareness to raising (lots) of money for cancer research. Lance has since created his own three-ring binder, the Livestrong survivor notebook; it helps with practical details like financial planning and treatment record keeping and shares survivor stories. It's available on the LAF website and online bookstores. This is champion work from Lance and everyone in the community owes him an incredible thanks. Lance is routinely on television occupying his new role as a survivor and inspiring others to beat cancer like him. His impact is worldwide and sustained; he's our community's finest ambassador.

I'd like to extend Lance's theme to the obligation of those still fighting and the obligation of those who lost. While the lucky ones who have beaten this disease do have something to teach, the rest of us may have even more to offer.

Our family friend, Judy, died last year after battling cancer for more than 20 years. She was never able to declare total victory like Lance but in between recurrences, repeat surgeries and new rounds of chemotherapy, she watched her children grow, go to college, get married and have children of their own. It was a recurring battle for Judy but she lived a wonderful life. Judy looked beautiful at Thomas Sweets, the classic ice cream shop on Nassau Street in Princeton, NJ. We were both bald from our treatments, Judy with a floral bandanna and me with a baseball cap. We smiled at each other while the generations of our families squealed and jostled for their blend-ins and cones. She was dying but out having a great time and being a role model for me. Judy understood her obligation as a fighter to live life with grace and to keep fighting even when you're losing. She was gone a few months after our ice cream adventure but still always present for me. I have a sense Judy was fulfilling her obligation as a fighter.

Nancy is my childhood friend's mother. As adolescent boys, her son, Keith, would bristle when we voted his the "hottest mom." A schoolteacher for decades, Nancy is a few years past what Google gave her for odds. Her ovarian cancer spread and in between road trips to her grandchildren and dream vacations to the old country, Nancy has pulled out tumors that have spread everywhere including to her brain. Nancy remains active, positive and happy. Never a quitter, after 5 years battling, Nancy is in full remission! She has looked after her son's friend offering encouragement and support; I believe her example has made an enormous difference.

Effie is my mother-in-law; she beat breast cancer in the 1980s and recently a new cancer took out the roof of her mouth. It's hard on her because everything having to do with eating is difficult and when you're a Taiwanese-American, everything is about eating! Effie carries on; she is touring Yellowstone Park as I write this chapter and insists on living life and moving forward. This is in spite of losing her husband, Jim, to cancer a year before I got sick. Jim was strong and healthy at 72, as fit as a man could be. A pain at his side proved not to be an injury from the gym but colon cancer and he was gone very quickly with grace, dignity and honor. I learned immensely from both. I also learned immensely from Bernice, my rock of a wife, who buried her father and supported her husband and mother as we all entered Cancerville simultaneously.

The ones that are still fighting and the ones that lost have taught me about the obligation of the fighter. I received boxes of letters when I fell ill from people at the phone company where I worked, many of them with sick spouses, parents and children. It's good for people to see celebrity athletes, rock stars and famous actors take on this disease. But after watching Judy, Nancy, Effie and Jim, I felt a special obligation to comport myself with dignity and offer the people in my cancer community a *mortal* role model.

After getting the all clear from my doctor 21 days after my last round of chemo, I put on a suit and went back to work the next day. There was a large team meeting and I was called up on stage and welcomed back from my misery. I still had the sickly pallor from chemo and the odd baldness amplified by having no eyebrows or facial hair. I was puffy and swollen and looked something like an over-plump hotdog stuffed into a suit. I grabbed the microphone, told them it was a gift to be alive and a gift to work, and thanked them for their encouragement and support. I've been humbled by how many people are looking at me as a source of encouragement for the battle they are fighting. So many have stopped by or sent an email telling me how they've used my story as encouragement to their husband or son. Lance is on the global stage; I don't know how he does it. It scares me to death just being a symbol in my tiny corner of Cancerville.

I hope I comport myself well and I hope I don't let these people down by dying. If I do die, I hope I can do it with dignity and grace like Judy and Jim.

# 14_____

# One Year (not) Wiser

It's been a year now; my hair is back and except for the surgical scar, I look and feel relatively normal. If you approach me from my good side, you'd have no idea about the trauma I endured and the battle I fought.

I shelved the idea of writing this book for a long time; it was time to live again, not wallow in my cancer story. It was a good year most of the time. I've reconnected with friends, travelled with the family and started to rebuild somewhat of a normal life. I've concentrated on getting fit and am spending a lot of time on the exercise bike.

Work is very different now. I haven't changed the "professional Scott" very much but the interesting thing is they all have changed. Being a cancer patient has simplified things. People seem to understand I have none of the usual workplace political motives; a guy fighting cancer isn't busy trying to undermine some rival department. They take me on face value and seem to see me as a more independent arbiter of truth during the many conflicts that plague corporate life. I still call things like I see them and still am the same pushy, opinionated, influencer that I always was. Since cancer, it seems to play differently.

With the benefit of some distance, I've re-opened the "Word" document and re-read the book I had started. I'm not sure why. I threw out the first chapters and reworked things; it was all too dark and no longer representative of my mindset. The book changed from being therapeutic and cathartic, something written mainly for me, to being something I hoped could serve the community and last for my family. My kids are 10 and 8 now and I thought about writing something I would be proud for them to read. I have a thousand scraps, chapters started, others discarded. Sometimes I wonder if there is something wrong with me thinking I can write a book. There are a million cancer patients; do I really have something to say? Maybe it's a "chemo-brain" delusion.

I might be writing again because I'm not really ok. I have another scan in a few weeks and I don't feel right. My eye is twitching, there's pain behind it and I have a pain in the back of my head—all surgical side symptoms. I know my "scanxiety" tendencies, but at nighttime when I try to sleep, I'm sure the monster is back. I'm feeling stressed about it and my blood pressure is high. I know it's why I restarted the book after closing it all those months.

I'm not really present even when I'm there at the dinner table, watching Gavin's baseball practice or driving Zoe to her play date. I'm obsessing. Joyous times with my kids have turned depressing as I can't help but picture these recitals and ball games without me. I'm having trouble at happy events. Birthdays and holidays are melancholy for me. Will it be my last? Something about these holidays makes me take stock and reflect. I'm supposed to be having fun but I can't. A few weeks to go before another scan; will the bubble burst?

# 15

## Saint Marcolini

It is summertime, 2009. Another year passed. I'm still alive 40 months after surgery and I've started, stopped and revised this book a hundred times. My body has recovered and my mood and mind are much better now most of the time. I still obsess immediately before scans but I'm generally ok until 30 days before the next check. My scans are now every 6 months instead of every 90 days so with half the scans, I have half the stress!

There's been a lot of stress though in the last two years. I found a small bump on the white of my surgical side eye; I had deep bone pain in my leg; I found a hard nodule on the palm of my hand; the lymph node on my neck under the surgical scar was swollen and hard; muscles in my face on the surgical side suddenly started to twitch as did my eye and then it started on the other side too; I developed a dry cough without any cold symptoms; my neck started to feel constricted as if a belt was pulled tight around it; my thyroid became swollen and tingled;

and I developed severe acid reflux and burning in my throat and esophagus. I know, it's quite a list (and quite a sentence).

Each of these events created incredible anxiety for me and required me to wait for the next scan—usually a month or two away before getting any resolution. Because of unclear results, even after the scans, I had to endure other procedures to rule out cancer recurrence. That meant an ultrasound of my thyroid, a colonoscopy and endoscopy, blood work and dedicated scans to specific trouble spots. It's been quite an up and down ride. Still, I'm developing perspective; amazingly, all of that turned out to be ok. I've gone many rounds with cancer and I'm still standing.

I made a mistake last month and brought scanxiety to my friend Andy's wedding. Logistics made me schedule my scans a day after his special day. It was a risky environment for me: long-lost friends, a few drinks, toasts to good friends who are gone…it all got a bit too heavy for me. It was a wedding; when people asked me how I was doing, I shouldn't have told them! I was a little too open about my struggle and confessed to being nervous about upcoming scans. Sorry dear friends! I shared a bit too much; especially with how well things were going. It was six months since the previous scan and it was the most symptom-free, uneventful interval between scans ever. Everything had been going pretty well and I was strangely calm and peaceful.

I took the morning train from Princeton Junction to New York and got my PET and whole body CT done at the MSKCC main hospital. I was more relaxed this time. Everything was smooth. The train was right on time and a subway car arrived as soon as I hit the platform. I got to the hospital without any stress and with time to spare. Green lights the entire way!

I felt a new sense of belonging on this trip. I had become an old pro and the entire staff seemed to know me. I felt I had earned some frequent flyer points. My instincts were sharp; I could tell immediately when a nurse entered the room if she would be able to find a vein. It's something about the way she carries herself that gives her away. I give them two tries before I request a new nurse; once they miss twice they're flustered and can't do it. They're usually grateful for the reprieve. Experience matters.

I drank the Crystal Light contrast solution for the scan and this time, during a position change for the PET, I asked if I could take a bathroom break. Why not? I was a regular customer, why was I suffering discomfort; I probably paid for half the radiology wing, why not take a few privileges? It took me three years to have the bravery to question authority like that. Why hadn't I done that before?

Before the sickening iodine injection went in, I told the nurse that I hate it and nearly always throw up. Surprised, she offered to adjust the speed of the drip to let it in more gradually and it went off without a hitch; not even a hint of nausea. Why did I not ask before?

This was the best trip ever. All of my demons were being vanquished and it was smooth sailing. I was finally in charge, a champion in the ring with cancer on the ropes. I felt like a veteran, experienced and worthy to be in the fight; finally calling some shots, taking charge of my situation, and feeling comfortable in my skin.

After a day off, I was back in the city to get a head and neck CT in midtown. Sudden panic struck on the uptown E train. Was I getting too cocky? Had I let my guard down? Why was I so calm? I was a day away from another "open door moment!" I scolded myself for not keeping up the vigil. I was totally unprepared for bad news and I was superstitious that I would somehow let it in if I didn't stay on guard.

The fifth floor suite at MSKCC's 53rd Street facility was packed to capacity like always. My blood pressure was high and had been climbing steadily throughout the day. I'd been here so many times before. It was my open door appointment, an office visit to hear about the results of my scans. My doctor didn't call this time to give me the good news; he made me come in to talk about it. I worried that meant bad news was coming. Maybe I shouldn't have let my guard down. I was on time and checked in at 3:45 but the doctor was running an hour late as usual. I sat down and felt my blood pressure climb again as I waited for another life-altering verdict.

"Oh my God!" Something horrible occurred to me. I checked and rechecked my backpack but it wasn't there. I've had 16 open door moments and 16 times the results were good and 16 times I "rewarded" my doctor with a box of Belgian chocolates. In my rush to the city, I left the chocolates at home. Was this an omen? On my most carefree trip with my most positive mindset, wouldn't it be ironic if number 17, the time without the chocolates, was the time it all unraveled? I was too cocky. I broke my own rules. I made this trip alone with no listener advocate to join me. I forgot my system of celebrating and rewarding the community. I could feel the pressure rising in my veins. I was alone, unprepared and facing the open door.

While I awaited my verdict, Lance was racing again, out of retirement and in the hunt for another victory on the final few legs of the Tour. It seemed like destiny my verdict coming at the same moment as Lance's triumphant comeback tour. Maybe it all had been a tease. For a while there, I started thinking maybe I was like Lance, a hero like him who beat the odds. I should never have deluded myself like that. I'm not Lance. I'm a mortal human being with anxiety, superstition, insecurity and doubt. I'm not a hero or a survivor. I'm just hanging on and hoping. I'm half the man Lance Armstrong is and always will be. Sure, I had made it longer than I thought I could, but winners like Lance close the deal; "almost" doesn't count in world championship competitions.

I picked up my BlackBerry to call Bernice, I needed to let out my emotion and tell her it was all about to go bad. But instead, I opened my web browser. I Googled Marcolini chocolates and saw there was a store in midtown on Park Avenue about ten blocks away. If the doctor was late like always, I could just make it there and back in time; ridiculous superstition, something Lance would never do. I decided to forget it, the report was written; it was already on the doctor's desk. It couldn't make a difference now. The ink wouldn't re-form and write itself into new words if I bought a box of chocolate.

Reception called my name and like usual I was brought from the comfortable lounge back to the office area and waited alone in a cold and sterile examination room. The doctor was getting closer. He was probably just reading the scan reports now for the first time. I could hear his voice beyond the door talking to other patients and his staff. He was making rounds. 15 minutes, then 30 went by and my stress reached a boiling point.

I had heard it 16 times before. It was the same knock as always, two quick raps from the knuckles and a turn of the handle. It was my open door moment. I craned my neck around the door to try to get a look at his face. I could see it in his eyes immediately; he was all smiles, he had both thumbs up. Deep sighs and laughs. My blood pressure shot down in an instant; like one of those air mattresses after you pull the plug. He told me I looked good and I told him I felt good. We chatted for awhile and shook hands. We made a date to see each other again around Christmas. He turned to leave and I stopped him. I opened my pack and handed him the small black box, fresh from a roundtrip sprint to Park Avenue. "Don't forget these," I said. "Remember, you keep giving me good news and I keep giving you Belgium's finest chocolates".

Later that week I heard the news. Lance finished his comeback race at the Tour de France, short of victory, but in a respectable third place. "Maybe he's just human," I smiled to myself, "and maybe I've got a little bit of Lance in me after all." Maybe all of us mortals do.

**Please Support the Liddy Shriver Sarcoma Initiative**

The mission of the Liddy Shriver Sarcoma Initiative is to improve the quality of life for people dealing with sarcoma. The Initiative increases public awareness of sarcoma, raises funds to award research grants, and provides support and timely information to sarcoma patients, their families, and medical professionals. These efforts are achieved through collaboration with numerous individuals and organizations that share a similar vision.

Visit the initiative at
http://sarcomahelp.org/

Proceeds from this book will be donated to the "Initiative"

# Endnotes

1. The Lance Armstrong Performance Program ISBN 1-57954-270-0

2. BMJ, October 17, 1998. "Cancer Diagnosis is Often Missed."
   http://www.bmj.com/cgi/content/extract/317/7165/1033/a

3. Sydney Morning Herald, June 2008. "Fighting Spirit Won't Beat Cancer."
   http://www.smh.com.au/lifestyle/wellbeing/fighting-spirit-wont-beat-cancer-20090407-9xm4.html

4. Dr. Kathleen M. Foley, "Why is Cancer Painful?"
   http://abcnews.go.com/Health/CommonPainProblems

5. Oncology Nursing Congress Survey, 1999.

6. National Cancer Institute. SEER Cancer Statistics Review 1975-2006

7. Period of life Table, U.S. Social Security Administration 2005.
   http://www.ssa.gov/OACT/STATS/table4c6.html

8. Global Policy Forum.
   http://www.globalpolicy.org/component/content/article/109/27519.html

9. American Cancer Society. "Effects of Supplements on Treatment.
   http://www.cancer.org/docroot/mbc/content/mbc_6_2x_herbs_vitamins_minerals_supplements_and_antioxidants.asp

10. USC News, February 5, 2009. "Green Tea Blocks Benefit of Cancer Drug."

11. Cancer Weekly, May 7 2002. "St John's Wort Weakens Cancer Drug"

12. University of Maryland Medical Center. "Green Tea".
    http://www.umm.edu/altmed/articles/green-tea-000255.htm

Made in the USA
Lexington, KY
09 November 2015